If They Tell You You're Dying…
Bring Something To Do (Ray's Last Words)

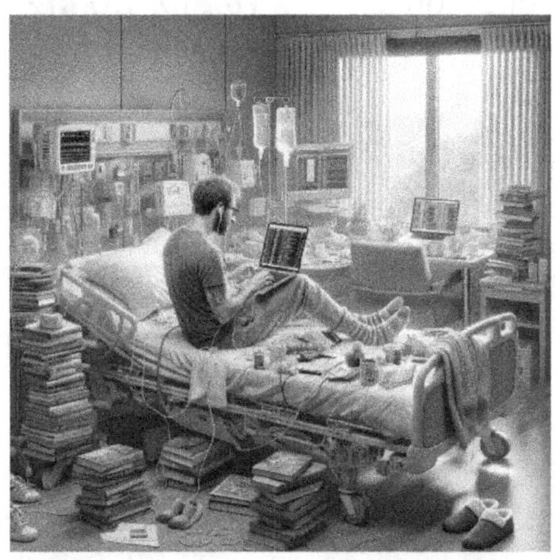

By RAY CHARLES GORDON

***Cover Art by DALL-E via OpenAI ChatGPT-4**

Foreword

"While I waited [for Ty Cobb to die]: Ernest Hemingway blew his brains out, Getty bought Honolulu Oil, Coke came out in cans, and the brunette in the courtyard ran away with a handsome young lawyer, and on July 17, 1961, Ty Cobb died quietly in his sleep." – ***Cobb*** (1994)

Most people have all the right answers to all the wrong questions. Story selection is the worst bias, and the answer to one-quarter of all question is "***f**k you for asking***."

Introduction:
What I Do Whenever I Have Nothing Else To Do

Had I quit chess when diagnosed with end-stage liver disease in June, 2021, I would never have ***solved chess*** (in theory), nor published a nearly-perfect, narrow, ***complete*** repertoire in a mere twenty-five pages, accompanied by all my other books (PDF), games (PGN), and digital opening repertoire (CTG), serving notice to my opponents that, as with Mike Tyson, knowing what's coming won't help.

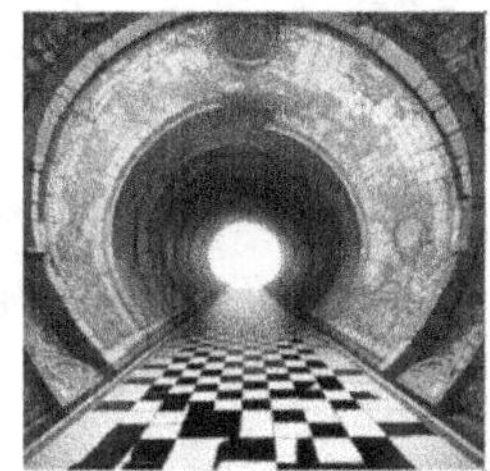

The chessplayer who can force a draw from move one, like Kramnik did with the ***Berlin Wall*** to swipe Kasparov's title in 2000, will easily dominate the chess world, usually by winning due to the opponent's impatience, poor technique, or attempting to force a win when none exists. Chess engines made the ***tunnel*** repertoire possible, and on August 20, 2023, I put it to the test at the ***Main Line Chess And Games*** monthly quads, a surprisingly strong regional Sunday morning event which attracts many prodigies, led by Tariq Yue, whose rapid rise from 1200 in early 2021, at age seven, to just under 2000 (1991) when paired against me in round one, in my second live tournament of the year and third since 2017, with my rating (now 1787) well off its peak of 2000 in 1989, at age twenty-two. Everyone knew what would happen: the rising star would easily dispatch the dinosaur, likely with superior opening play.

Four hours earlier, I awoke in my Chinatown loft, to a warm, late-summer Sunday morning, still functional enough – ***barely*** – to make the trip to the tournament if I wanted, but playing online would have been <u>***so***</u> much easier. Still, I knew there would be prodigies, and was eager to get a rematch against one I had drawn at my previous quad there, and in a filler game at the Philadelphia Open. Instead, I was served up to the young lion, who politely said ***maybe*** when I asked if he was the "top five something or other in the country." His reputation preceded him. At fifty-six, I viewed live, tournament chess (itself rendered obsolete by online play) as Jack Lengyel did Marshall football in 1971: it wasn't whether I won or lost, or even how I played the game, but ***that*** I played the game, that I was still able to rise, dress, groom, pack a bag, ride forty miles on SEPTA in a bathroom-free car to Paoli, climb a steep hill to get to the venue, and sit down for two hours to play not checkers in a nursing home, but a highly relevant game of chess against a future champion, on whose career I would have an extremely minor influence.

This alone was something money couldn't buy, and which a ***nest egg*** tends to preclude. Aside from the obvious generational clash of players on opposite trajectories, I was just a stepping stone, another fiftysomething Class-A player with some good stories, and hopelessly outclassed in the opening, with a brain that can no longer learn new tricks. Worse yet, I was an ***online one-minute*** player, meaning I'd fall apart at a slow time control, and be unable to handle the precision required for OTB tournament play, especially against this youngster. Yue played like the well-schooled prodigies on scholarship at Dalton in the 1980s, canonized by Fred Waitzkin in *Searching For Bobby Fischer,* which I might have titled *If Your Son Plays Tournament Chess, Bring Something To Do,* since he whittled away the several hours he spent at the first Sunday New Jersey quads in Somerset, a bustling chess event which attracted the best prodigies of the day, many of whom would go on to fame, fortune and power.

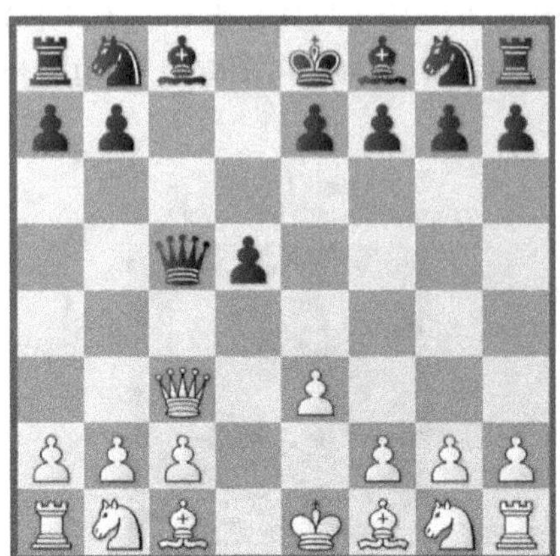

Moves: 1 e3 d5 2 d4 c5 3 Qa5+ Qd2! 4 Qxc5 Qc3!!

This opening – a reversed Queen's Gambit Accepted (QGA) in a line that easily forces a draw through early queen liquidation – did not occur in the game, as Yue had White and played an accelerated fianchetto system for which I was well prepared, but had yet to *solve*, meaning I would have to – <*gasp!*> -- actually *think* six or seven moves into the game, instead of the fifteen to twenty in lines like the Rubenstein French or QGA, the latter of which I used to defeat 42nd-ranked GM Anton Korobov in 2019 in a one-minute game on ICC, two years before he beat Kasparov *twice* in a blitz tournament, to avoid becoming best known for losing to me! I almost quit after that game, figuring I'd never top it, but I was about to be proven wrong, tossed into the most ferocious chess battle of my life against a mini-Karpov and potential *future world champion*, much like I would have been had Dad preferred chess clubs to arcades and racetracks or OTB parlors, where my youthful Saturdays were spent.

Somehow, I swiped the initiative in the opening, relying on general knowledge and specific preparation in similar lines. I almost never emerge from the opening with an inferior position, and held the edge here, until a key move where he could have won a pawn but perhaps lost a piece, or the initiative, and I've never checked the engines to find out. My guess is he could have beaten me, but that was his only chance. After declining my challenge, Yue made two positional errors, first giving me a bishop pair by doubling my pawns and allowing me to force an exchange that gave me a protected passed pawn supported by the Bishop pair, which cost him a piece for one pawn, not the easiest of positions to win. Move by move, I consolidated, snuffed out his edge, then forced him into an exchange of rooks which let me mop up as his flag finally fell. His tenacity, and ability to remain composed even when getting *b******pped* by Black, impressed me. Soon after, a 14-2 run kicked Yue's rating up another seventy-five points, and he remains in the top five for age ten. I took his autograph on my scoresheet as I thanked him for the game.

Imagine being able to shut down Steph Curry in his prime, or to toss a complete-game shutout in Major League Baseball, and now imagine doing this at *fifty-six*! This single win reestablished me as a serious tournament player, and caused other prodigies, parents, and coaches to take notice. In a world where prodigies are coached by true dinosaurs, who marry their ratings by ceasing tournament play so they can cash in by teaching obsolete theory, I went into battle and prevailed against one of their actual opponents, and best of all, I proved to myself that I could actually make the trip, as well as proving that my brain was still sharp. When attempting to place a value on the equivalent nest egg, I couldn't find one, though I suspect I'd trade this exhilarating, *life-affirming* experience for perhaps a cool half-million that the healthcare system would immediately cannibalize, given my condition, and the ***Estate Recovery Act,*** which collects repayment from the estate for all Medicaid costs incurred after age fifty-five. By contrast, I played a game of chess which could be replayed in perpetuity, long after I'm gone.

Just shy of my twentieth birthday, I made training at chess what I would do whenever I had nothing else to do, and six months shy of my twenty-fifth birthday, I quit tournament play, having failed to secure the Samford Fellowship while eligible. I kept playing against legendary hustler Tom "Murph" Murphy, a blitz champion (World Open 2005) who was recently in a McDonald's commercial, and who wins tournaments as a senior citizen (he's one of the top five blitz players in America among seniors), to keep my game tuned, as I patiently waited…and ***waited…***for the engines to solve the game, so I could copy what they did into the tunnel. I had expected this to occur no later than 2003, but it was not until 2019 or so that the silicon became strong enough to seed the tunnel, a clear example of how timing is as important as talent or effort: what I did against Yue, and in the eight years leading up, was simply not possible in the 1990s, when I elected not to waste my time on a board game only to wind up tenth or fifteenth in the world. Now, however, I have finally hit my stride, for as many strides as I have left.

* * *

Money is that jerk who controls your life, dictating where and with whom you should hang out, enslaving you as its protector, making you cling to it for dear life, having convinced you that you cannot live without it, at the cost of your spirituality, your very soul, and all those *loser* activities, like chess, or watching sports, or gambling, which will leave you destitute in old age. ***Tell me you don't know how Social Security works without telling me…***while it is no longer true that the elderly and infirm are not dying on the streets ***en masse***, our system protects almost everyone, especially the elderly and infirm, not to pass judgment on those who have truly hit bottom. Yet another use of my waiting-to-die time has been to intensify my advocacy for the homeless, at a time when society is more receptive than ever. I have already facilitated some major changes in housing laws, though I never took proper credit. Suffice it to say that when you tweet a good idea to someone in power, as a *rando*, they are more than happy to steal it. This was not intentional, just a byproduct of censorship.

While I can never completely rule out becoming world champion, at my age that is no longer necessary to establish a legacy, as my progress since 2015, and especially 2019, attests, and I am not yet done improving. With that said, the knowledge that I might only progress from my 2337 one-minute peak on LiChess (equivalent to 2150-2200 FIDE) to say 2500, leaves me wondering if it is worth overcoming ***the law of diminishing returns***, as few would notice the difference, but I continue training in my spare time because *I* would, as would the future generations who build upon my work. Those who have only a six-figure nest egg that will soon vanish due to illness will never know the thrill of having improved the life of another like this.

The win over Yue was the product of a lifetime devoted to maximizing productivity, including times where I was unemployed or otherwise idled. By training as intensely as possible during these times, I was able to accumulate an impressive body of chess knowledge that has propelled me to a lifetime peak (online) rating at age *fifty-seven*, when most of my age peers are several hundred points below their glory days. This suggests that had I continued playing in my twenties and beyond, I might have reached the pinnacle, but I was not willing to gamble my best years on this, particularly since chess makes for a perfect retirement activity (it's about all I can do anymore at a high level), while *pickup artistry* has no senior division.

Those who think old guys with money make out like bandits need only look at the *#metoo* lawsuits to realize just how *inferior* these men are viewed by women. One reason I built my life around getting laid in my twenties is that men in their thirties and forties, and *especially* their fifties, rarely get laid on anything but *sexwork* terms, which my prime precludes me from ever considering. Now throw in social media, where women make seven figures off PG-13 content, and you get a *sexual dust bowl* where most men are *#incel*, and women live behind a paywall. My PUA days are long, long gone, leaving me undistracted by things like popularity, or *mobility*, which are anathema to the rising young star of a game not really worth the time of anyone capable of solving it. It has long been rumored that Carl Schlecter could easily have defeated Emmanuel Lasker in 1910 for the world title, but that it did not pay enough.

Chess is not my only unexpected retirement benefit. Indeed, just about every "waste of time" from those twenties I maximized has taken center stage in retirement, leaving me occupied literally every waking moment, with productive, influential, and sometimes *profitable* activities greatly enhanced by the strong foundation laid over three decades ago. I found this surprising, as I had bought into the *financial-security* narrative, perpetuated almost entirely by women who seek to trade sex for said security, leaving a generation of *#mgtow* men learning this the hard way; indeed, to admit one's wife is a glorified hooker is to admit that one is a John. In my prime, my intelligence, intensive study of women and conscious effort to become attractive to them, and earning potential made my finances, or even *living with my mother* irrelevant, but at my age I acknowledge the role of money and gifts in "game," unapologetically, for numerous reasons, though this renders women more of a luxury than a necessity.

When I am not playing chess, my days are filled with sports betting, daily fantasy sports (DFS), and daytrading (usually *SPY* or *SPX* options), but not horse racing, due to the horrific deaths of Maple Leaf Mel and New York Thunder in 2023, or I'd have yet another time-consuming repository from my youth, one which I had actually curtailed except for big days due to rebated whale bettors, except on big days, but now I refuse to even watch the animal torture posing as sport. Female company is as easy to find as ever – my last two girlfriends were nineteen and twenty, just a few years ago, but took up so much of my time I had to end the relationships. One more peak performance with the opposite sex would be a nice way to go out, though my existing memories are more than sufficient.

Small Minds Talk About People

As an early internet adapter, I experienced online haters, threats, doxing, harassment, defamation, unfair business competition, plagiarism, and a host of other ills which only now are becoming known to the masses. Sadly, search engines and their immunity from lawsuits have caused a lot of the garbage content to remain accessible to anyone who has your name. On the upside, the advent of video, the use of real names, and most people existing entirely online, with haters who put mine to shame, as well as my advanced age and no longer being much of a threat to anyone, efforts to "cancel" me tend to achieve little, particularly since anyone in my condition gets priority for rescue from the government. While my disability check originally stemmed from being blacklisted as a whistleblower from office work, my physical condition ensures I'll likely remain retired until the end. Though well below average, subsidies and budgeting have allowed me to get this far, with the occasional windfall from trading or betting, and the ongoing threat to break the bank at any time, something I've already done on a small scale.

Once upon a time, I filed a series of lawsuits over internet defamation and harassment, as well as separate employment discrimination complaints against the University of Pennsylvania, which I'll discuss later. To make a very *tl;dr* story short, an internet personality who reminds me of Bixby Snider from *Robocop* put me on blast in front of an audience of 2,000, with the goal of causing a "tilt." Insults flowed, but the last one stood out: ***"You'll never accomplish anything with chess."*** At this moment, I had an epiphany: with just a few years left on this earth, I could spend my time engulfed in timewasting internet drama, or I could continue to channel my energy into chess, further developing my legacy. Whatever time I had left would no longer be wasted. It also became clear that this is how celebrities deal with haters: make art consumed by the world, and ignore the noise.

Years ago, I did a popular YouTube video about how secondary benefits make a smaller social security check larger than a bigger one, and another about how one should not save a cent for retirement, beliefs which have been confirmed by the past few years. While I never had a nest egg, my ***whisability*** at age forty-eight allowed me to enjoy a decent fraction of my time with financial stability that was elusive in my youth, in turn allowing my chessgame and other endeavors to thrive. This text also brings my number of published titles since my diagnosis to around half a dozen. Meanwhile, "Bixby" has thrived, in a ***Jerry Springer*** kind of way, inviting controversy which dwarfs what landed me briefly in his disgusting universe. I am much prouder of this legacy than I ever would have been with anything involving people like them or any hater. My fan base, while small, is more intelligent and loyal than anything anyone, including me, deserves.

With my first "terminal" diagnosis of stage III COPD in 2002, which included a prediction that I would not survive, the decade, I sit here twenty-two years later with a pulse-ox that rose back to the mid-90s from 83 in 2005, only to begin dropping as the ***ascites*** from my end-stage liver disease compromises my insides, and Type II diabetes continues its methodical destruction of my endocrine system, with blood-sugar numbers which panic doctors, yet which are not fatal until much higher, when ***diabetic keto acidosis*** kicks in, as it did on the Saturday I spent in the Jefferson ER the day Jeffrey Epstein died, learning much more than I cared to know. Despite this, I am completely functional intellectually, even as I rapidly decline physically, my body preserving its core functions.

As some point, my health will give way, but not without more than enough time to finish this text, train some more at chess (no need to play live ever again as I proved I could do so at a high level), and spend most of my days doing not only what I love, but what is now the ideal activity for my situation: ***day-trading 0dte SPX options!!*** With long-term planning completely out the window, what would normally be clinically insane money management can be embraced, as can high-stakes sports betting, and even short-term flings with women (more later).

Your Time Portfolio

In subsequent chapters I will detail how none of the above is an accident, but rather the ***payoff*** from sound investments of my ***time*** in my youth, which has ***compounded*** over time to catapult me to a lifetime peak chess rating, and the ability to turn a very small amount of money into a very large amount of money in a ***very short period of time***, the latter of which is critical to anyone facing terminal illness. With that said, liver disease makes me much more ***fragile*** than sick, and I awaken most mornings able to at least make it to my desk and make YouTube videos, play chess, trade, or bet, and when the urge strikes, the weather is good, and I've just gone to the bathroom (so I don't have to while in transit), I can still pack my things for a forty-mile day trip to Paoli, or a hundred-mile trip to the Marshall, the latter hosting a nifty under-2000 Saturday morning tournament where I had my first 2-0 start in over thirty years, before blundering away a $94.75 prize, in another life-affirming road trip.

Loudmouthed, verbally aggressive, self-asserted experts like I was in 1998 with the PUA community, tend to dominate the internet, with video and streaming making sexuality and popularity the most valuable commodities, as evidenced by the seven-figure incomes of top quasi-adult models. Since I no longer desire to compete in such a jungle, I have mostly retreated into obscurity, save for my online videos and writing, instead focusing on chess, trading, betting, and coding bots that might one day break the bank, and which almost already have several times. I know of few wealthy elderly who truly enjoy life in a way that doesn't require large expenditures and the exploitation of the working class, all the while pretending they are actually liked for something other than their finances.

Even if you are already in retirement, you still have ***time*** to accomplish ***something***. I cannot live your life for you, only share my own experience and let the reader do what they will. I wrote this text primarily to kill time, but also as a final summary of a life I have already bored the world with in print far too many times. ***Outfoxing The Foxes (1998)*** was written not because I wanted to be an author, but because I grew tired of answering the same questions repeatedly, and had eight hours a night to kill during third shift at the concierge desk in my building, where I made $6.00 an hour, originally while training at chess, and later coding and writing. My gambling books were internal documentation of profitable methods in case something happened to me, including how to operate my bots, while my chess books were my training material and playbook, later converted for a public audience who found value in the method I used to reach 2337 at one-minute on LiChess, and 2000 USCF back in 1989.

Put much more simply, I was a lot like Kramer from ***Seinfeld.*** Michael Richards said he used to play Kramer as if he were a step behind everyone, then began playing him as if he were one step ahead, making the character what he is known for today, what might be called a ***sigma male***.

One:
I Got The Horse Right Here (Intellectual Dishonesty)

The stereotypical ***basic bitch*** is both intellectually dishonest and manipulated by others just like them, building entire lives on lies, falsehoods, and often deliberate misdirection. If you ***do what you love*** expecting the money to follow, but not really caring because ***money doesn't matter***, since ***women like nice guys*** and the ***best man wins*** (because your favorite television character told you), then ***you got this!*** If the homeless bother you too much, you can vote for politicians who will get them ***the help they need***, which you know will occur in a humane setting, even if you've never seen the place for yourself, while you count on the tooth fairy to pay the $10,000.00 a week to care for a single vagrant who could have been housed instead for $500.00 a month. You ***know*** you're right because *everyone* (in your echo chamber) tells you that you are, and anyone who thinks otherwise is a bitter, whining, loser, hater, and mentally-ill ***#incel*** who needs therapy!

Anyone who still wonders why I interact primarily with chess, AI, and my betting bots should read the above paragraph again, preferably several times. By giving everyone a voice, we create ***false equivalence*** between right and wrong, good and bad, smart and stupid, and truth and lies, evolving into a groupthink narrative enforced by your ***social credit score***. Like most, in my youth I was blind to this carcinogen, allowing others to shape my beliefs, reality, and even my ***future*** with lies, misinformation, or simple ignorance they would impose on me as if something were wrong with me if I didn't agree. What I should have questioned, but didn't, was why ***my*** life choices mattered to ***them***. As I learned with age, only young, attractive, smart, and well-off people are doted upon this way, by social-climbers who want a piece of the action for themselves, or to build themselves up by tearing down others.

Idiocracy warned of the dumbing-down of humanity, but those folks were well-intentioned; Intellectual dishonesty adds malice. Sealioning and gaslighting are extreme examples, but it is what flies under the radar which quietly destroys us, all by design. One example is the "common knowledge that ***all hypnosis is self-hypnosis***, which means that anyone who claims to be raped or molested by a hypnotist ***must be lying***, all the while the hypnopredators – many of whom perform on-stage at "dry" prom and grad nights – operate in plain sight, completely unscathed. That I received death threats when I warned of this, as well as doxing, harassment, and audience manipulation by skilled practitioners, should makes one wonder which nerve I had struck. That people can have major surgery without anesthesia under hypnosis should (but doesn't) put to rest the claim that anything you can do with hypnosis, you can do without.

The more I succeeded at anything, the more intense the gaslighting: ***not a master by twenty-one, never a champion*** was used to dismiss any notion that I might have world chess championship potential even at twenty, with funding and hype directed at the prodigies who never made it, usually quitting once they came of age. ***Wait for the right woman*** made me passive towards finding love and sex, a mistake corrected in 1991 when I began thinking for myself, and learning from one of the best PUAs in the world for an entire summer. All of these pale in comparison, however, to what those who told me ***don't listen to other people*** would throw a tantrum over when I took that advice to ignore their warning that ***you can't beat the races***, or ***you can beat a race, but YOU CAN'T BEAT THE RACES.*** The unbridled hostility inherent in being singled out for a reminder that what you have been doing your entire life is simply not possible – implying I was a ***liar*** if I claimed otherwise – was designed to ***gaslight*** me either into going on tilt and losing, or not betting. The more I ignored this advice, the more intense the abuse, usually from people who are the first to ask for the wealth to be spread when I won.

This was not specific to horse racing. In college, I had an impromptu, three-hour "dinner date" with a new crush late one Sunday afternoon, only to learn a few days later, from a friend of my best friend, that she was ***out of my league***. At the time I politely endured the advice, only to figure out later on that she had rejected all of them the previous semester, prior to my arrival, and they could not accept my success with her, itself the result of years of hard work figuring out how to attract the world's sexiest women, since it challenged their world view that my lifestyle was inferior. Fortunately, Dad had trained me to be an independent thinker, and by *dying* in 1979, cleared my path for an independent lifestyle which increasingly annoyed others who had no reason to care how I lived, yet did, particularly with regard to horse racing. This came to a head in 1986, when those who wished me well after I dropped out of SUNY/Albany, while facing eviction from a three-bedroom, rent-stabilized apartment, suddenly turned red with envy when learning that I was doing a little ***too*** well at the track.

Compounding Your Interests

For all the advice about compound interest growing your financial nest egg, ***compounding your interests*** does the same for your hobbies: devote your entire life to something for which you have talent, and in old age you'll have much more than just a way to pass your final days, as you continue to build on a robust foundation. As with your financial nest egg, the more you ***invest*** in your hobbies in your youth, the greater the compounding effect, resulting in the difference between being fifty-six and enjoying a nice game of chess in the park, and being fifty-six and defeating one of the most promising juniors in America. The racetrack is full of retirees who meticulously budget their leftover fixed income for a $2.00 bet each race, but it's the legends like Bill Benter and Andrew Beyer who remained relevant and influential later in life, because they had a stronger foundation on which to build. The process of building that foundation, however, requires a leap of faith in one's youth that few are willing to take.

As it turned out, the deaths of Maple Leaf Mel and New York Thunder at Saratoga in 2023 caused me to cease horseplaying, but the sport could just as easily have filled my retirement with meaningful entertainment, and an equally meaningful chance of breaking the bank, all thanks to Dad's training and then Mom's and my own continuation of the incredible foundation he laid. All of this was lost on society, however, which didn't hesitate to brand me a degenerate, at which point verbal abuse was warranted, lest anyone else consider stepping out of line. The ***odds*** of any gambler throwing caution to the wind to study high-level theory and risk all of one's time and money to pull off what Beyer did are slim, particularly given the social pressure against doing so, pressure which becomes increasingly overt if you might actually succeed, as I learned in 1986, after dropping out.

My family has a long history with horse racing and gambling, most of it a cautionary tale. My SHBaunt (SHB = ***Smoking Hot Babe*** in #pua lingo) owned Cockey Miss, a stakeswinning juvenile at Monmouth in 1967, and runnerup to Eclipse Award winning Queen of the Stage. Unfortunately, she married a compulsive gambler who cost her the horse, her mail order fortune, and East End Bowl (80th and York), my future hangout, before he moved on to prison, and she to the afterlife, courtesy of cirrhosis taking its final toll at age forty-three, without warning, the surprise call coming in to Mom one Sunday night in 1977. Despite this, and despite Dad and half my family on each side dying of liver disease, I never heeded the warning, spending my life drinking enough to have died years ago.

Mom was very familiar with the track, but only through tagging along with my Aunt or Dad, and was particularly fond of Santa Anita and Del Mar, which they frequented while Dad was on business in West Hollywood, where I was born in 1967, before they moved back to the UES (Eighty-Ninth and First) in 1969, where I recall dangling from a tenth-floor window before Mom moved us to the second floor of the skyscraper in which I grew up, after which she ceased participation in the family pastime. Dad, on the other hand, began schooling me on the intricacies of harness racing and its betting, in a manner more commonly associated with developing a chess prodigy.

By age ten, I dazzled my summer camp counselors with my handicapping knowledge, setting the table for a lifetime of growth which, were it not for the equine atrocities, would still be paying dividends now. Instead, it serves more as a lesson in intellectual dishonesty, uniquely qualified to bring out the worst, and dumbest, in the masses. The mere *mention* of horseplaying causes all kinds of reactions, most of them negative, often triggering lectures against compulsive gambling and degeneracy, followed by ostracization by people I never tried to win over in the first place. Our tendency for approval-seeking winds up letting the intellectual dishonesty of others dictate our lives. The same could also be said for cutting school, for which I was looked down upon by teachers who saw me walking with Mom during lunch, yet who remained silent about the *bullying* which drove me to learn more from sitcom reruns than my textbooks.

To excel at the track, which makes for a more enjoyable retirement, you need the type of head start rare in any field, such as chess, but even rarer at the track, since children are not supposed to wager at all. In my childhood, I ran into a few likeminded young strays at the OTB or track, most of whom were chasing easy money, and had nothing to offer as handicappers, but the exceptions were notable, leading to by far the best friendships of my life, though it also attracted some degenerate slime, like the man who moved in with the mother of one of my wealthy neighbors, with them blissfully unaware or willfully blind to his ways. Dad, on the other hand, was a *sharp horseplayer*, often winning large amounts of money, some of which I witnessed, but also losing, as I learned upon discovery of a camp locker packed with losing bets, not collected for tax purposes, but including his favorite "lucky number" combinations. Dad was a good handicapper, but so was *Degenerate John*.

On April 1, 1980, a month before I would barely squeak through eighth grade with a high fever during finals, I returned from a two-week sabbatical (cutting) to an assembly, blissfully unaware of the date. The mock *career day* recited all the options other than college, inspired by the many trade-school commercials which aired during the day. The *gambling* skit, of course, mentioned two "graduates" from the school: me, and a future NTRA handicapping champion. Apparently, our reputations preceded us, and not in a good way. Also apparently, the head start that his parents allowed and mine engineered resulted in each of us winning substantial money over our lives, a literal fortune in his case. When I noted after the assembly that these were viable career options, the teachers laughed, continuing to mock me, which I thought about during the financial crisis of 2008, another event that independent thinkers saw coming but to which the public ignored, because no buzzwords warned them.

At thirteen, I was already an experienced horseplayer who had *beaten the races* for seven straight years, raising the ire of anyone who learned of this, prompting anything from disdain to outright verbal abuse, or in this case, public humiliation of a kind that today would get the adults fired or sued. What stood out to me, however, was the baldfaced *elitism* in a place on the fringes of the prep school circuit, even more so after a midyear move from Fifty-Fourth and Fifth to Eighty-Third and Amsterdam, where

I got mugged within a month by kids from Sammy "The Bull" Gravano's alma mater (the *600* school), and where I had my first kiss, on the median at Eighty-Third and Broadway. Decades later, I learned about my peers from that first kiss, with whom I didn't have time to hang out, because I was working for Mom, but this didn't stop them from looking down on me as a "lowly gambler" even if I was working.

Horse racing was an integral part of my childhood, thanks to Dad's lifetime passion for gambling, and a high income ($50,000.00+ a year in the 1970s) which allowed him to spend his evenings doping out winners at Roosevelt and Yonkers. His mission to make me *hustle-proof* had me learning every game under the sun, including poker, but it was the trips to the track or the OTB at Eighty-Seventh and Third (near *Papaya King,* for whom sold franchises) that I remember most about our brief coexistence. Fifty-nine when he died in 1979, Mom was twenty years his junior, having met him in 1964 on a quickie mail-order product called *Memory Treasures*, introduced by an uncle just after the Kennedy assassination, who made millions when he wasn't in prison for mail fraud relating to advertising; Dad also spent a year in *Club Fed* for something similar. Here's a brief highlight film:

- The first race I ever watched was Secretariat's thirty-one length, triple-crown clinching win in the Belmont Stakes, at Dad's insistence that I not miss *history*, for which I am grateful in retrospect. This race made clear that some horses are simply faster than others.

- My first recollection of harness racing was on a Saturday afternoon card at Roosevelt in 1973, followed by a number of trips where I was taught *trip handicapping*, pace, cover (wind), being parked wide, and Dad's favorite *double move* (three-wide) angle, on the theory that the driver was trying to win, and that the horse will win "off the move." On my ninth birthday, I used this angle to hit a $6.00 win bet on a 21-1 shot that keyed a $1,200.00 trifecta (triple) for Dad, who doubled my allowance in perpetuity rather than giving me all my winnings at once.

- Our Saturday routine was pretty standard (for us): a visit to *Playland* at 50th and Seventh, near the OTB where Dad would bet the thoroughbreds, followed by a ride up to *Papaya King,* where he'd conduct his franchise business while sitting me down at the Eighty-Seventh Street store. After cutting ties with former franchisee Nicholas Gray, who went on to found *Gray's Papaya*, Dad was called in to recruit new franchisees, though only one store opened briefly at Fifty-Sixth and Lexington before closing shortly before Dad died. I did get twenty-two free hotdogs as a thanks for writing an ad, and looked forward to watching the races on Channel 9 at 11:30 p.m. Giving in to the temptation to call the OTB result line before the broadcast meant having to keep a poker face, which usually failed. If Yonkers was running, we'd often go there.

- On Christmas Eve, 1974, Dad returned home during a driving snowstorm to inform our cash-poor family (recession) that he had lost at Yonkers. I asked if he had bet 4-8-6 (DHF) in the tenth at *Monticello*, which hadn't run yet, and he said no, after which he got in his leased Oldsmobile, drove back to the OTB in a driving snowstorm, and returned a few hours later with the after-tax proceeds of a $2,400.00+ trifecta hit (about $1,800.00). "*Santa*" would later spend all night testing the *Pachinko* machine he left me the next morning.

- When Dad died in 1979, I quit cold turkey, save for getting tossed out of the OTB parlor (with the future NTRA champion), and did not look back, instead throwing myself into Manhattan life during the summer, which included a regrettable month of day camp. With my new ten-speed, I began doing messenger work for Mom at minimum wage ($3.35 an hour), while still collecting an allowance that would stop in 1980, and experienced the thrill of spending my paycheck, often on

Beef Satae with Peanut Sauce at the ***Bangkok House***, next door to the legendary comedy club ***Catch A Rising Star***.

Like the opening in chess, childhood has the greatest influence on our lives by virtue of being first. The ***trajectory*** Dad had set for me had turned me into a hardcore, ***compulsive*** gambler, because while gambling is addictive to some, though never to me, ***winning*** is addictive to everyone, flipping the script to where ***not*** betting cost money. Winning at chess also prompted me to continue with the game, good enough to ***beat my friends***, at the time thought to be just a shade weaker than Fischer, who just had much stronger friends that I could learn to beat. Today, of course, one can be rated online in minutes.

Both of my parents were ***hustlers*** and remote workers before it was fashionable. Our dining room/third bedroom became Mom's office, with each of our ***six*** telephone lines dedicated to her business, or one of Dad's franchise projects. Their favorite sayings were ***we're not poor, we're broke***, and ***your ability to make money is your savings.*** This kept me sharp, but it also kept me without that all-important ***nest egg***, which meant I would die broke on the streets in old age, something easily avoidable, if only I'd put down that ***Racing Form***, take school more seriously, finish college, and get a high-paying job on Wall Street or in Midtown, for one of Mom's ***Fortune 500*** and celebrity clientele. At ten, I had to keep the ***Time Man of the Year*** secret, in between off-hour calls in search of anyone open, while at thirteen, I was picking up tapes and delivering transcripts to NYSSA, with all of Wall Street grinding to a halt until I arrived at 71 Wall Street on my bicycle. My home had a photocopier.

Much like a newborn given stock in a growth industry, my time portfolio began to explode, especially after Mom took me and my anti-gambling SHBCousin to the 1980 Belmont Stakes, won by Temperence Hill ($108.80), who she briefly liked before showing gender solidarity with runnerup Genuine Risk. Having been bit by the gambling bug, my very opportunistic mother decided that I "missed" the racetrack (I didn't), which led to biweekly excursions (weekly was "too degenerate") to the second-floor Clubhouse dining room at Belmont, and later Aqueduct, once racing finished at Saratoga. Bribed with a $30.00 bankroll, which I multiplied on six of our seven trips, and free lunch, Mom had herself the free selections from the ***math-prodigy*** tout Dad had so meticulously developed.,

Prodigy or not, without the many years of hard work that went into my training, I would have been just another racetrack rando, wasting time instead of very inadvertently building a retirement weapon. Without question, I was enjoying the present, but according to ***them*** (the omnipotent group who runs everything), I would pay the price in old age, and for my entire adult life, for all the time I was "wasting." Few are those who continue to ignore such social pressure, all rooted in the intellectual dishonesty of someone who cares not about your well-being, but who feels threatened by anyone with the potential to leapfrog them socioeconomically in the 1:10.2 or thereabouts that it takes to win a six-furlong stakes race.

<u>Pick Your Own Horses</u>

Excellent advice for anyone, yet Dad never thought to liberate Mom from piggybacking his "expert" selections and wagers, with her content to remain a passive participant. On Saturday, November 1, 1980, our seventh mother-son bonding trip, this time to Aqueduct, via the only Mercedes taxicab in the city (a surprisingly low $12.00 fare!), Mom began asking me who I liked, prompting me to walk downstairs, purchase a second ***Racing Form***, place it in front of her, with an advisory to pick her own horses, and advice to consider jockeys and workouts, with twelve seconds per furlong considered good speed. After Gentleman Jinsky ($28.80) took the second, and Smug ($20.00) took the sixth, with two other pricey winners rounding out the card, her $5.00 win/show bets left her $400.00+ to the good, memorialized by the *New York Times* results page taped to her nightstand, with all four winners circled, a stunning blow for feminism and against Dad's patriarchal ways.

Mom quickly proved that her big win was anything but beginner's luck, as her exploits far exceeded Dad's, with biweekly trips to the track giving way to daily excursions to either UES OTB (the other one at Sixty-Ninth and Second), and any midtown or downtown parlors which coincided with her shopping and other errands, most often to Fifty-Eighth and Lexington, due to proximity to *Alexander's* and *Bloomingdales*, her two favorite shops, conveniently situated near the M-31, which ran almost to our doorstep. Saturdays were usually spent at the Beach Café, which still stands at Seventieth and Second, apparently a favorite venue for dealmakers and venture capitalists. While I liked the food, I spent more time in the *McDonald's* across the street, or playing videogames at the *7-11* next door. Around the block was a bookie joint where I bought my first football cards, where ties lost, and every spread was a key number; somehow, I still showed a profit.

For all my alleged degeneracy, my peers weren't exactly lighting the world on fire, except for my former classmate Cynthia Nixon, who took up acting as a way of making money. Most of my friends just played sports or arcade games, hung out, watched television, and stumbled through school. Horseplaying and chess were *mindbuilding* exercises that yield time and sometimes financial dividends to this day, yet each is considered a colossal waste of time or money for adults, a bit less so after *The Queen's Gambit*. Bobby Fischer was viewed as living on the fringes of society even as he ascended to the world championship! For those who deemed me the *next Fischer,* he had become a cautionary tale more than a role model. The decision to become a gambler was made for me as a toddler, specifically because Dad wanted me to have as many financial weapons as possible, and to make me immune to hustlers and ruin; he succeeded, but in doing so, addicted me to winning; bless his soul.

<u>Strike Three</u>

Mom's revival of my horseplaying interrupted my increasing patronage of Met and Yankee games, where my knack for nabbing foul balls in batting practice fueled many sandlot games at Fifty-Ninth and A, softball in the Wagner schoolyard, riding my bicycle, doing messenger work (about $225.00 a week as I was now paid by the package), and living the good life. My combined Christmas/birthday present of a season ticket to the 1981 Mets had me positioned for playoff tickets once they finished building their dynasty, likely shortly after Darryl Strawberry was called up. Unfortunately, my ticket was refunded, and later abandoned, thanks to the Baseball Strike of 1981, which punctured my hero-worship of these ingrateful, overpaid prima donnas, leaving me with no alternatives to the track, into which I had thrown myself with *Ainslie's Complete Guide To Thoroughbred Racing*, the "horseplayer's bible."

The *Spring of Fourteen* had me on "sabbatical," due to Rhodes informing me that I had already flunked the year, and would have to attend summer school, but I chose instead to repeat the year, as I was on track to graduate at seventeen and wanted to be a legal adult while away at college (I wouldn't get any studying done in Manhattan). This led to working fulltime for Mom, betting at OTB and the track, mostly through her due to my age, winning $200.00 on a gift $5.00 late double from John The Super (who had a thing for Mom), for a lesson in trainer moves, and most importantly, a chance meeting with Scott, a/k/a ***Banned4Life,*** a seventeen year-old dropout who had just gotten his GED, while working as a messenger for Mobile, Mom's former service prior to my swiping the contract.

Banned introduced me to modern handicapping theory: Beyer, Davidowitz (Dad had a copy of ***Betting Thoroughbreds*** in the bathroom but I didn't understand it at nine), and Quirin, among others, were covered. We mocked touts like Mike Warren, who sold a handicapping system based on pace that didn't sound too bad, but were most intrigued by ***My $50,000.00 Year At The Races***, Beyer's followup to ***Picking Winners***. In another example of compounding one's interests, Beyer would win millions many years later, long after publication of his golden goose, and reflect on how ***little*** he bet during this time, in a game ***they*** say cannot be beaten. Maybe ***they*** couldn't beat the game, but Beyer sure could, even publishing the very playbook he was using to do it. At some point, I would have to try this method.

The ***Summer of Fourteen*** was a mélange of OTB, messenger work, skating all over the city, and the harness tracks in the evening. A few days prior to the 1981 Belmont, I called into CNN and asked John Campo, trainer of triple-crown hopeful Pleasant Colony, if he thought Summing ($16.00) might steal the race. ***"Never been done,"*** he replied, ignoring that Bold Forbes had done just that in 1976. As it turned out, I had only a $1.00 "souvenir" bet on Pleasant Colony (a likely worthless digital ticket), due to the sloppy track, and my ***$310.00*** win on the OTB late double at Yonkers, a blind pool with a 2-1 and 14-1 winner paying triple the parlay, a lesson on compounding winners without extra takeout.

Long before retirement, my compounding interest in horseracing was yielding substantial tangible rewards, in this case enough to cover a month's bills, all the while earning me the rightful scorn of anyone who saw my ***Racing Form***, including my maternal grandmother, who expressed disapproval on my visit to Mary Manning Walsh. Mom's side of the family had grown substantially wealthier than when she picked up their pieces after her sister and brother-in-law died in a plane crash in 1966, and of course she had to pitch in by caring for their teenagers for an entire summer. Those teens had grown into highly successful adults, while I was ***<u>wasting my life at OTB</u>***; no further exploration of my life was necessary to condemn me as a degenerate gambler and threat to the well-being of those around me.

Just before Labor Day, 1981, I was ***Banned4Life*** from NYRA, or so I was told by the ***age police***, who found me minutes after a waitress in the dining room chewed me out for leaving a $1.75 tip on an $8.25 lunch check. I cried my way home through a distant part of Queens, resigned to playing harness tracks or OTB for my remaining years, only to wind up released back into the wild at Aqueduct a few months later after tossing a snowball at Angel Cordero, Jr. in the winner's circle (his horse beat mine). I realized then that ***no one really gives a f**k*** about anyone or anything; I was told the lie in the hope they'd keep me away for a little while, which they did. On Labor Day, while at a Mets game, I picked up $170.00 on the Fall Highweight Handicap, an indication that my studying with Banned (including ten days in his Mom's apartment after she moved) was paying off. Now six feet tall, and always on skates, I was finally able to place my own wagers.

Three weeks after Labor Day – September 26, 1981, to be exact – I skated to the payphone near the Band Shell, after bailing on an overcrowded free concert from Simon & Garfunkel, to check on my trifecta (triple) wagers I had doped out at McDonald's that morning, placing them at OTB before embarking on my day. I had boxed A-B-I, tossing the K at the last minute, cutting my box from $24.00 to $6.00. With the sweaty ticket in my pocket, I learned to take better care of my tickets, but also that the K nosed the A for third, costing me a $3,600.00+ trifecta, and serving notice that I was capable of hitting jackpot bets. I was encouraged, but also stuck at *Wagner*, six blocks from OTB, with mandatory attendance precluding weekday play, and just about everything else I had enjoyed for nine months. Bored, and tired of my peer group, I walked out on Friday, November 20, 1981, never to look back.

Too Cool For School

An hour after leaving Wagner, and a half-hour after we rejected enrolling me directly in Hunter College to preserve my Social Security Death Benefit through age twenty-two, I landed in the ***Quintano's School For Young Professionals***, which had graduated three of my cousins, soon to be four, and which served as an academic refuge for slackers, would-be-dropouts, and working actors or models, which is how my cousin hooked up with Diane Lane for three years (they didn't hide this so there's no need for me to either). Within two months, an impromptu walk out of school led to my second kiss, first date, and a relationship that did not end until our last date just before I moved in 1986. School was perfectly situated within a quarter-mile of five OTB parlors, and right next to the A train, a straight shot to Aqueduct, and a transfer away from the E and F to 179th Street, Jamaica, followed by a ride on the N6, which let me arrive in time for the third or fourth on most school days.

Late 1981 was when the compounding interest in horse racing began to pay off:

♦ An hour after enrolling at Quintano's, Mom and I won ***$380.00+*** at OTB, prompting the jealous teller to note that my age was showing as Mom collected (they knew I was underage and let me bet anyway). The next afternoon, we went to the Meadowlands, where I won another $60.00.

♦ On Saturday, December 19, 1981, I took $20.00 earmarked for the Jet game the next day, put $10.00 to win on Thirty Eight Paces ($9.60), who won the Gravesend Handicap by nine lengths, and a $10.00 late double ($36.60) with Hour of Love ($10.00), the horse who won us the $380.00 mentioned above, netting me $186.00 in profits, taxi rides to and from Shea, and an expensive lunch from a nearby deli (batter-fried chicken). Jet games were fun, but Shea wasn't built for football, and my interest in attending sporting events wound down as my love life picked up. These windfalls seemed perfectly normal to me, rare as they were for a teen.

♦ On Thursday, January 7, 1982, I used Beyer's speed-rating chart, without variants, to win $1,600.00+ on a trifecta (triple) wheel of a 7-1 winner over a 22-1 place horse. With the proceeds, I bought high-level custom skates, which I used to pick up a twenty-two year-old on Second Avenue on a bitterly cold Friday evening by outrunning the M-15 from Sixty-Eighth to Thirty-Fourth, with enough time to spare to change into my sneakers before she arrived. I settled for a makeout, and a week later, met my girlfriend. I did lose back $200.00 at Roosevelt that Saturday, the first of many signs it was time to leave harness racing behind, which I refused to do mostly out of loyalty to my training, an example of intellectual dishonesty to oneself, and very costly.

♦ Unbeknownst to me at the time, Beyer and Bill Benter, plus Ragozin and Brown with *The Sheets* and *Thorograph*, were decimating the NYRA pools, killing prices on the low-hanging fruit that sustained my ROI. By mid-1982, my winnings became more infrequent, but my streak had already ended after the weather shut down the inner dirt track for six weeks, my edge nowhere to be found. I continued to bet recreationally, but chose not to blow my winnings on an expensive computer, which I mistakenly thought I needed to make Beyer-method numbers (I didn't).

Money Follows Knowledge (The Rollup)

Recently, I did a YouTube video entitled ***Golddigging 101,*** about the three types of rich men:

- Those who cannot replace what they have;
- Those who have to work for what they have; and
- ***Those who can multiply money***.

The third category is the only true wealth, since the first makes one a slave to their nest egg, specifically the fear of losing it, to the point where it runs their life and guides their decisions, including to be financially selfish. High earners who have to work for what they have can replace their wealth, but only at a cost, and are limited in their ability to advance. It is the third category of men who, like Beyer and Benter, can rebuild from scratch, and are truly free of the risk of long-term ruin that sets in, particularly in old age, where the first two categories will not recover, while the third will. Those who have ***lectured*** me for my entire life about fiscal responsibility have all the right answers to all the wrong questions, the right question being who will recover fastest when a single illness in old age wipes them opt, making them more ***financially insecure*** than even me.

The ability to turn small amounts of money into large amounts of money in a short period of time – I call it a ***rollup*** – is the only true wealth, an expansion of Mom and Dad's central life thesis. Thanks to Dad, I already had this ability, and thanks to ***The Handicapper,*** Robert Kalich's fictionalized autobiography, I would add another weapon once I figured out how to make the ***power ratings*** that were central to protagonist "David Lazar's" journey from compulsive gambler forty dimes in debt to converting a $250.00 starting bankroll in 1970 into tens of millions in 1975, then many millions more until he retired in 2006, a year in which he picked ***74 percent*** winners, more than even a "scamdicapper" would claim. Just knowing this was ***<u>possible</u>*** changed my life, while most who preach financial stability never develop a shortcut to achieving that goal, while making them immune even to bankruptcy.

The Handicapper, set in Manhattan, offered a glimpse of my future, in much the same way as those mocked ***Playboy*** articles, written for single men who want to attract gorgeous women, long before the internet desensitized us to their presence. "David's" journey from degenerate ***loser*** walked out on by his wife, to conquering a nice corner of the world, became both my handicapping and life blueprint, marked by the endless pursuit of knowledge that I would hopefully one day convert into money, quite possibly overnight, while my haters chased a ***normal*** life of financial stability without jackpot potential. Compounding the issue was that horseplaying was conducted in public, with high visibility, almost ensuring a hit to one's reputation as someone who ***hangs out at the OTB,*** though far superior in my estimate to someone who judges others, inaccurately at that.

The many hours I spent exploring handicapping theory and methods, and the many more I whittled away at the cost-free hobby it yielded (Mom noted that the track was no more expensive than other entertainment, and she could come home with a profit), not even realizing the power of having broken even, as that gave me unlimited practice to further develop my edge. Those who admonish me for not saving for requirement wind up with little more than a pile of money destined for the healthcare system, and which they won't be able to enjoy as they could have in the youth they sacrificed to acquire it. For as nice as a regular job, income, or inherited wealth may be, my handicapping skill could never be taken from me, even – *especially* – in bankruptcy, while in my youth it filled many of my days and occasionally my pockets. That leaves me in a far better position in old age than if I'd never played.

Horseplaying gave way to school and socializing until the ***Spring of Sixteen,*** my last hurrah as a ***handicapping prodigy***:

- On May 3, 1983, I cut school by diverting to Port Authority after a messenger run for Mom. My *New York Post* horoscope said "count on good financial luck today," and I did, returning for the final four races for that reason, where I found a trifecta box ticket that I tried to cancel, couldn't, and which won on a disqualification after the leader knocked the second horse over the rail at the furlong pole. My 35-1, 50-1, and 14-1 shots paid ***$4,292.00***, of which I had half, for my best day ever at the races until 2009, which irked me no end, as it was mostly luck, though I had found several dozen tickets by kicking them over on the floor and memorizing the results.

- On Saturday, July 2, 1983, Au Point ($17.00), returning from having cut a fast pace in the Belmont (1:59.4 for ten furlongs around two turns, a tick off the one-turn track record), against much weaker opposition in the Dwyer. Mom bet $100.00, as did a few other friends, and half of the UES, it seems, as my ***pick of the century*** (like Fischer's ***Game of the Century)*** was 20-1 on the morning line, more likely hammered by pace handicappers, an area where my expertise was well beyond Beyer's, or just about anyone's.

- On Saturday, July 23, 1983, I had my first ***rollup***, turning my last $6.00 into $125.00 in the final four races at Belmont, which ended at 6:30 p.m., just long enough for the short ride to Roosevelt, where I had $50.00 on three-time winner and French champion Ideal du Gazeau ($11.00), who jogged home after being parked all five turns, bringing my bankroll to a cool $500.00 when I returned home after a fifteen-hour day "wasting time" doing what I loved most, particularly in the top rows of the fourth-floor grandstand, where Pinkertons feared to tread, and the winds blew the weed smoke away from the building through the back.

An incredible leap of faith is required to become a profitable bettor, since most of the money will be made at the very end, thanks to money following knowledge, and one will endure verbal abuse every step of the way from almost anyone who learns one is attempting to do the impossible and ***beat the races***, or the bookie, stock market, or any game which offers quick, "easy" money to those who conquer it. I had enough faith in my math skills and Dad's training to persevere even during lean times, and there were many, particularly after this streak. Save for a $100.00 place bet on Swale in the 1984 Belmont ($5.00 to win and $4.40 to place), I would not make a significant hit until early 1986, though I would have had Wild Again ($62.00) in the inaugural Breeders' Cup Classic, since his owners took 5-1 by paying $400,000.00 to supplement him into the race.

Most of my money that year ($3,000.00+) was made hustling bowling, but that ended when I aged out of the junior leagues. Almost all of it was made in pot games after the league, or against a rich preppy who initially attempted to ***gaslight*** me into thinking I couldn't possibly beat his power shot, which I learned had terrible control, and he was not the best spare-shooter, while I rarely left an open frame. Small-stakes games gave way to high-stakes, professional-style matches on a lane pair with alternating two-frame turns, and I always managed to hold sway, wondering why he didn't just give up. One Saturday in early 1984 I threw nineteen 200+ games out of twenty-one, and uncrumpled close to $1,000.00 in profits in front of my amazed peer group. A bicycle injury in Central Park ended my interest in a sport where every part of the body was vulnerable, plus I didn't like practicing.

The ***Spring of Seventeen*** was marked by unrequited love of my ***one true lust***, and the loss of my virginity on New York state primary night, at Gary Hart's campaign party at a Midtown hotel, followed by a summer spent volunteering for the Mondale campaign, which I quit after Reagan's age quip in the debate ended all hope. In between was a summer of chess instruction in Washington Square Park with Richard Gilmartin, with whom I'd grab a table just before ten, play for a few hours while smoking high-grade weed, buy him pizza, then return to the table to apply his lessons to my peers. By the end of the summer, I had developed a tournament-strength opening repertoire, and was estimated to play at around 1700 strength, before the weather got bad and college approached.

Women For Sale

My ***one true lust*** (OTL) was a fascinating young woman who ultimately rejected me because she "deserved the best in life," which I was unable to provide. This hit like a ton of bricks, leading to a half-hearted suicide attempt that preceded my post-convalescence emergence in the West Village. I also began taking manuscript work through Mom's service, expanding the family business, and a year later purchased a pair of IBM 95 memory typewriters to modernize, but was fighting a losing battle against word processing, whose incompatibility, as well as high salaries on Wall Street, destroyed Mom's freelance-heavy business model, leaving her with a core of clients that barely paid our rent. I hadn't realized that without horseplaying, we'd have already gone bankrupt, while the world concluded instead that we had fallen prey to compulsive gambling, making us pariahs, even within our own family.

College offered a fresh start, a quiet place to study, and a challenge to my plan of getting a 4.0 GPA in a business major, then going to Harvard Law on my way to a career on Wall Street as a constitutional lawyer, MBA, or combination of the two, at a six-figure starting salary that would have women like the OTL lining up around the block, requiring little more than financial security which, like any good prostitute, they would trade sex to obtain while being intellectually dishonest by pretending to love these men, and disparaging men like me under pretext, lest they appear like the golddigging hookers they more or less are, and which our intellectual dishonesty prohibits us from acknowledging.

At college, I would meet Kate, whose gift of the score from the musical ***Chess***, and her refusal to take so much as a dollar from me, altered my trajectory away from ***financial security*** and towards chess, on the belief that she was the canary in the ***sapiosexual*** coal mine, a signal, however counterintuitive, that ***chicks dig chessplayers***. I reasoned that by assuming the persona of ***The American***, I would attract many Kates, and not with ***financial security.***, If either Kate or the OTL had married me, I'd have ceased being the man who wrote this text, which I expressed in ***Bettor Off Single***, noting that women would not have tolerated the losing streaks long enough to hang around for the wins, as both Billy Walters and Robert Kalich learned firsthand right before they won their fortunes.

I hadn't even turned eighteen by the time I had a fully vested ***time portfolio*** that could easily both occupy and fund a nice retirement, without having to sacrifice my youth and beyond in an unfair exchange of my valuable time for money, time made valuable because I applied it to developing elite skills in multiple disciplines, though you really only need one, if at all. Even something as simple as <u>**woodworking**</u> could serve the same purpose, as could anything else that keeps one productively occupied, with a chance to make money, much easier now than it was in my day. This requires an expanded view of wealth, including your time portfolio and profit potential, rather than just your nest egg, which will be wiped out by a single illness in retirement, also triggering the ***Estate Recovery Act***, which forfeits to the government, from your estate, any money paid on your behalf by Medicaid after you turn fifty-five. You may very well wind up purchasing this text from Uncle Sam!

The Winning Horseplayer

Beyer's 1982 classic escaped my line of sight until a hungover trip to Crossgates Mall, in a futile attempt to replace a "double shot" glass broken at a finals party in my dorm the previous evening (I did get the host a nice set of four) had me stumbling past ***B. Dalton*** on the way out, with ***The Winning Horseplayer*** staring me in the face. Enthralled by the text, in which Beyer added trip and pace handicapping to his speed figures, I called Mom excitedly, asking her to save every day's ***Racing Form*** until my return, which she almost did, missing only three days, better than I expected. Mom shared that we were being evicted from our rent-stabilized apartment, due to an abusive boyfriend (that she met at OTB) modifying our apartment for his construction company, without written permission.

As a paralegal, I later learned enough to have kept the apartment, but even then I passed on taking over a rent-controlled apartment that would have been rent-stabilized two years later, and I did find excellent housing in Philadelphia, so I have few regrets, but to return home just shy of nineteen with nowhere to go, no job, and a bounced $2,004.00 check from Mom holding up my transcript (preventing a transfer), I never felt more alone in the world, yet I remained oddly calm. This was the perfect time to test Beyer's method, as I had wanted to do in January, 1982, one of the more expensive omissions of my life, given the limited shelf life of winning methods. A common mistake we make is to not get while the getting is good. I also took trip notes, which I had already done at Yonkers due to Dad's training.

Though I did hit a $50.00 win bet on Arctic Groom ($11.80) a week or so after returning home, ten days after the hit on Paul Castellano, in front of Sparks Steakhouse, near Grand Central, during rush hour, I scrambled together a working set of speed figures just after New Year's, igniting a nice, six-month ***staycation*** until I'd have to leave by July 15, 1986 (I wound up leaving ten days earlier after the Fourth of July centennial, or ***peak Reagan***, when I played chess all day in Washington Square Park for the last time). The highlight film shows how compounding took my time portfolio to the next level:

- The first day with the figures, I gave out two winners ($10.60 and $5.80), each of whom cruised by several lengths. Unfortunately, I ran out of money just as a big streak hit, but waited patiently for the next one, which came on Monday, January 20, 1986, when I took $15.00 I had earned typing a paper for a neighbor to Yonkers, tossing my last $3.00 on a cold 1-4-5 trifecta, horses I liked in the three most likely winning post positions. It paid $126.00, which I decided to use as a bankroll at Aqueduct, practicing ultra discipline, where I'd cut expenses to the bone, and wager $1.00 a race until I broke through, as my trip notes continued to accumulate. I neglected to notice that Beyer had a steady paycheck to tide him over during losing streaks, while I did not.

- After winning modestly for three days, on Saturday, January 25, 1986, I took the track bus ($3.50) from Fifty-Sixth, splurging a bit over my normal $1.50 subway commute (#6 train to 42nd, then the #4 to Fulton and the A to Aqueduct, with express trains home cutting the travel time in half), due to the rain, which made me decide to take only five jockeys all day: Cordero, Velazquez, Santagata, Davis, and Lovato. They would win all nine between them, including half of an $87.00 quinnella in the fourth, which gave me the money to take shots, half of a nice exacta in the seventh, and a $576.50 score in the finale on Mount Guard ($30.60), a clear figure play. I skipped home from Fifty-Third and Third in the rain, caught a cold, missed the next card, and deposited $750.00 in my bank account, expecting a great deal more.

♦ One afternoon, I caught Big McCoy ($12.00), a back-class longshot in the finale, with the $26.00 winner of the Eighth for a $262.00 double. Another day, I gave someone a four-horse trifecta box that won easily, making him a few hundred, and when he didn't thank me, gave him a five-horse box, which I didn't like as much, and lost. Other players would copy my figures, and a few white-collar types would drive me home for free. Unfortunately, I needed $50,000.00 a year in winnings to sustain my lifestyle, which meant I'd have to bet $120.00 a race, just to cover my living expenses while preserving my bankroll. My ROI for the meet was $1.17.

♦ Even after I quit in March, I continued to win, nailing Buck Aly ($20.00) over the statebred Landing Plot in the Bay Shore, for a $102.00 exacta two-and-a-half times, after scratching out a $20.00 wager at first. The maximum wager on the longest shot of the day, and four other winners, was still not enough to win the $25,000.00 handicapping tournament, in which I finished fourteenth. In May, having not seen a race in three weeks, I used the sheet to handicap, said *"Flunky Holme is 15-1?"* Mom wasn't impressed until he won, funding my final trip to Albany, for Spring Fling, in my old dorm room, where I got to say a proper goodbye to Kate. At home, I had my last date with my high school girlfriend, and then cut all ties.

I wound up winning several thousand dollars that spring, but should have won six figures or more. In March, I had a double exacta picked out, didn't play it, and it would have taken down a $70,000.00 pool, though "only" $50,000.00 after taxes, split between Mom and I, in New York City, so I needed more than just that, but it was symptomatic of my *disciplined* approach costing me money. On another day, a friend of Banned's stole $300.00 from his mother, which he lost at Belmont, while I took a borrowed $2.00, hit four races, and left with $117.00. Though I was losing my place to live, "Boards" (a wingman I had met at OTB), bankrolled me in a typing/typesetting business on the UPenn campus, and relocated me. I figured with a steady income and an edge, I did not have to rush. I was wrong.

Haterz Gonna H8

Taylor Swift, pardon the vernacular, is the queen of the basic bitch, who imagines herself held back by a cadre of *haters*, whose mere disdain somehow shackles her, particularly if she is attractive. It is true, however, that even a Swiftie can have genuine haters if her success annoys the wrong people, as mine at Aqueduct did, almost everywhere I turned:

♦ *My doormen* – two of whom used me to run bets since I fourteen –saw me leaving with my binoculars every morning, or coming back a winner most nights, with regular *Mahvelous Beef* from *Mrs. Tang's*, and the city's best bicycle-delivered weed, from an offshoot of the famous service. My confidence *bothered* them, though I was just trying to help some working guys win. They were having none of it, reminding me *you can't beat the races.*

♦ *Mom*, who took pride in her handicapping, was not a believer in *figures*, and didn't think I should be betting so much given that I hadn't seen a NYRA race other than the Belmont since 1983. The pressure of eviction was wearing more on her than me, though she initially turned down Philadelphia, instead trying to make it go at a women's residence on Fifty-Seventh Street similar to the Martha Washington house in *Bosom Buddies*, before caving in and joining me in my one-bedroom apartment in September, my independent wings clipped briefly; Mom would move out in October, 1986, and I would join her a year later, in March, 1987, in a tall building near UPenn.

- ♦ ***My (alleged) friends.*** I was already known as a ***degenerate gambler*** to my peers, and the neighborhood at large, but once I began paying my bills (***sans rent*** until July) with winnings, shades of ***envious green*** emerged, all couched in "helpful advice" not to ruin my life any more than losing my apartment had caused. That the apartment was gone before I made my first wager in ***three years***, taking Mom's once-great transcription service with it, was lost on everyone.

- ♦ ***My relatives.*** Thanks to my uncle's history of compulsive gambling, that side of the family did try to help, but gave up on us after a few months, given that Manhattan was a financial black hole. Mom could easily have gotten a high-paying job, but she was too proud and too burned out from things having fallen apart. She could have taken roommates after I left, but wasn't comfortable with that. That Mom had helped to raise orphans who happened to be blood seemed long ago, in a different world, but we all remained on good terms, especially once we stabilized in the mid-Atlantic, nearer to one of Mom's remaining sisters (three had died by 1984, two in their forties of cirrhosis and a third of a plane crash).

- ♦ ***My typing clients.*** Early 1986 brought clientele from all walks of life. I was pulling in a few hundred a week, which kept the lights on, while Mom and I made $25,000.00+ off a form-letter job where I had both IBM 95s running as I typed on the other. I treated the staycation as a test of Beyer's method, when I should have done the very simple math that said I had to be wagering $120.00 a race, when I was barely comfortable risking twenty. Over time, I became much better at exploiting my edge, but my patience cost me my place to live, landing me on the UPenn campus, while I was college age, in an area with literally tens of thousands of single women my age. Life wasn't so bad after all! Nevertheless, one fashion client chewed me out for thinking I could get rich at the track, advising me to seek office work, but no one was even interviewing men like me.

One Headlight

On the upside, my friends were more than happy to cash in, particularly Boards, who rolled $2.00 into ***$500.00*** on the last four races one Sunday. I won when I needed to, but since I was leaving town, and knew I would keep winning in the mid-Atlantic, I was more interested in tying up loose ends, which I did, catching up with my high school girlfriend, Kate, and everyone else. Banned drove up on the Fourth, in a dying car with literally one headlight, whose engine wouldn't start again if allowed to rest, and which was rolled into a makeshift spot at the edge of a garage, in a rainstorm, for a minor miracle. The next night, he drove me a hundred miles in a driving rainstorm, somehow keeping it running long enough to also make it home to Asbury Park, after getting me where I truly needed to go. I remained clueless about the meaning of ***bridge-and-tunnel*** until I used the latter to exit the city for good.

After a slow summer in Houston Hall, the "resume crush" netted me thousands of dollars in September, but changes in the resume-book rules nuked our typesetting revenue, leaving us with expensive, outdated equipment which sunk the business, leaving Mom to retreat to our new apartment in the Fairfax (Forty-Third and Locust, a gentrifying block) for typing clients, which barely kept us afloat. Worse yet, the mid-Atlantic tracks (particularly Garden State Park) did not offer the steady profits I had found at the NYRA tracks, sending me reeling. The concierge desk in the Fairfax offered a lifeline, and a discounted rent that gave us an even better deal than we had in New York. More importantly, it gave us breathing room, after a tumultuous period that shattered my privilege, but which also woke me up, in many ways the best thing that ever happened to me, in a ***redpill*** way.

By 1989, I had figured out how to win at Philadelphia Park, adding trainers and removing trip handicapping from my approach, resulting in tens of thousands of dollars in wins until the ***Beyer Armageddon*** in 1992, when the ***Racing Form*** began publishing his figures for all to see. The desk job was critical in both stabilizing my finances, and giving me a job at which I was encouraged to bring something to do, usually training at chess or handicapping. After 1991, I wouldn't win again until 1999, when I wrote ***How To Break Even At The Track,*** and the next decade was my strongest ever, in large part because the legal climate made sports betting impossible; at least the track was legal and paid off. In 2006, I won money I still haven't finished counting, all thanks to a seven-percent rebate from Pinnacle, the world's largest online sportsbook at the time.

Once I lost my rebates, along with my mother and Banned, in a six-month period in 2007, I lost my profitability, and reason to make horseplaying a priority, though its value in my time portfolio remained, particularly since my ***PAP*** method (***Price And Probability***) allowed me to hunt for jackpots. My last hurrah was in 2009, when I turned $20.00+ into $8,000.00+ in two weeks, but then conditions changed and I never locked in. As a jackpot hunter, I tend to risk any winnings in search of a big score, so breaking even or a slight loss is the best I can do. Unfortunately, in 2023, after watching Maple Leaf Mel and New York Thunder go down, not in battle like Ruffian, but cruising to the wire on broken bodies, I lost not my profitability, but my stomach.

More Haterz Gonna H8

My 1991 haters at the Center City Turf Club – a small, overcrowded theater box in Center City – put my 1986 haters to shame. They included:

- ***Staff.*** Not all, but a few were not thrilled to see me celebrating my wins, which was difficult to hide, since I was betting on my lunch hour and during breaks.

- ***Other horseplayers***. Physical threats from a few jealous patrons were par for the course back then, with the staff turning a blind eye. Much like any OTB, close quarters for gambling degenerates, many of whom are losing money they don't have, is not recommended. The internet age has eliminated the ***slime factor***, and I couldn't be happier. In 1990, however, I was just as happy when the Turf Club opened, since it saved me trips to the track to make ***PhoneBet*** deposits and withdrawals, even if I watched the races on ***Philadelphia Park Live***.

- ***My Boss.*** My worst hater of all was my boss, the late Sol Sardinsky, CPA, a horrible racist whose abuse I endured for a full year, inspired by Jackie Robinson's orders not to fight back, in order to establish ***resume stability***. Not long before I was mysteriously ***Banned4Life*** from the Turf Club (rescinded in 1998), I took a phone call from one of the managers there, who had asked for Sol. I had made the fatal mistake of sharing that while he was in New York City, I won ***$1,200.00*** on races I bet through PhoneBet and listened to on the phone with Mom, hoping he'd like that I didn't need a raise. Taking breaks didn't bother him, as women did this all the time for much longer, but the idea that I could become richer than him, or rich enough to leave, was intolerable, since he was effectively funding it. Two days after my first anniversary, with no raise, I left for a job at UPenn.

With regard to retirement planning, the track was offering me a way out of my gender-bias rut, the true source of my financial instability. Women my age were now earning $50,000.00+ a year, while I was making $18,500.00 to start, raised to $19,300.00, for Sol. The amount of money ***stolen*** by gender bias, all motivated by ***#metoo*** violations in an era where the "woke" were comatose, was impossible to recover. Men, especially *financially secure,* white-collar types, always ignored this truth while lecturing me on how to properly handle money, including not gambling it. My chess rule *never listen to your opponent* applies equally here, as these very same people put me in the position of seeking alternative paths – today they call it a *side hustle*. Additionally, I still had my freelancing, and the concierge desk as strong mitigators.

The 1991 haters were just a grown-up version of what I'd been dealing with my entire life. Without horseplaying, I never would have seen this side of people, who *perniciously* attempt to undermine my success with *soft-bashing*, or "negging," just enough of an insult to get the point across, while attempting to disguise it as helpful advice or even praise. In 1987, a teller at Garden State told me I was "wasting my life" at the track, yet never made clear why she was in my business in the first place, though when she married another "professional horseplayer" who I knew was a complete degenerate, and had three of his babies, it made sense. Horseplaying, and chess, had me doing temp work that masked the gender bias that was ripping my financial guts out. If I was going to improve financially, let alone save for retirement, it wasn't going to be through office work.

My First PUA Bootcamp

TrustFundDude was a fascinating pickup artist: literally unstoppable with women, and *independently wealthy…*sort of. A trust in his name worth $175,000.00 yielded enough to fund his $1,500.00 a month allowance, from which he paid his bills, and rationed the rest to fund his PUA lifestyle, into which I was integrated in June, 1991 after a chance meeting in the lobby. Very quickly, we fell into a routine of exchanging my horseplaying knowledge for his advice with women, while we would hit on them in pairs, or at times without their knowing we knew each other, to compare notes (he won that contest 8-1-1 and sabotaged me with the super-elite who wanted me over him, *gaslighting* me by telling me she didn't). By the end of summer, I had seen a side of women I wished I hadn't, and thought becoming a "dating expert" sounded better than "secretary" when asked what I did for work.

Not only had my horseplaying been profitable, it had opened doors both in business and now PUA, allowing me to make valuable, life-altering connections with people who benefitted as much from knowing me as I did them. It also cost me my rent-stabilized apartment, but only because we had to interact with the crowds. From the mid-1990s, it has been possible to wager from home, but back then the track was a centerpiece of American sport and leisure, resulting in much higher status for a sharp handicapper than now. While I have made similarly valuable connections through chess, I certainly wasn't making them through *work*, where I dealt with the worst of the worst *basic bitches*, a price I was not willing to pay just to achieve phantom security in an old age which would erase any nest egg once my health deteriorated. Freedom from this concern allowed me to *frontload* my lifestyle, or what they call *maximizing my twenties,* and not saving for retirement, long before doing so was fashionable.

High-Intensity Bodybuilding

By the end of the summer 1991 "bootcamp," I had developed a rather extensive body of PUA theory, most notably CUPID, a measure of *sexual market value* (SMV) a concept publicized in Academia, and mainstreamed in *Black And Single,* by Larry E. Davis, albeit with a subjective formula which I standardized (see *Bettor Off Single* or *Outfoxing The Foxes* on Kindle for more info). Once horseplaying became unprofitable, my lunch hours were spent at bookstores, perusing everything dating-advice book I could find. By 1994, I had read almost everything on the market, and had developed my own ideas, which included my *meal management system* for weight loss, which I combined with *High-Intensity Bodybuilding* by Ellington Darden, to lose forty-two pounds in eighteen weeks, achieving the best shape of my life, and proving once and for all that looks, youth, intelligence, and being *ripped AF* are worth infinitely more with women than "game," which was much easier to build with opportunity.

Darden's work is a fascinating study in intellectual dishonesty, not from him, but from a profit-driven fitness industry that favors complex, expensive solutions to Darden's simplistic approach, the latter rewarding independent thinkers like me with bodies like his, something I had failed to achieve for years of working half my body on alternating days, and doing endless repetitions that never seemed to do anything other than prevent me from getting fat, even then having failed me (obviously). Darden's advice was an epiphany of the kind I hope the reader has here:

- *Work the entire body at once*. Darden noted that it was unnatural to work only half the body during each session; I noted that this meant I'd be going to the gym three days a week instead of seven, later reduced to *two*.

- *Work each muscle to failure*, in as few reps as possible. "You don't become a better writer by repeatedly writing your name" was Darden's excellent analogy. Suddenly, instead of working multiple sets of each exercise, split over two days, my entire circuit took ninety minutes in one.

For another example of what money cannot buy, one Saturday morning I went back into the *Market West Athletic Club* to retrieve my jacket, only to find in the rear of the locker room mirror a naked, fat, old, *multimillionaire* Sol Sardinsky staring at me while I was in literally perfect shape. The striking contrast was noted in a frozen-in-time moment most men will never experience while they're busy making money and building a nest egg, and can't be bothered to trim the fat where it counts. *Why did I need wealth if I was attracting the sexiest women*? Money was nice, but to find a lover, all I had to do was walk outside, plus I had several other sapiosexual options left over from the chess world. If the goal of financial security was to become more appealing to women, I had already accomplished that, though money has uses far beyond getting laid. For retirement, I still seemed screwed.

The chance encounter with Sol was one of many convincers that chasing money was not the answer, that my high SMV was true wealth, but also that it had a definite shelf life. Making what seemed like a deal with the devil, I simply ignored all long-term financial planning, hoping to somehow score a jackpot. I never came close to achieving this, but was investing my *time* in a manner as sound as my finances were unsound. I may have been broke, and *living with mom*, but I already had "lucrative" retirement hobbies and an artist's persona that was getting me laid like gangbusters in the present. I blocked out any concerns that I would die broke, freeing me to live as I chose.

For all his flaws, Sol met the minimum standard for an acceptable employer, and he enabled my *resume stability*, but the best thing he did for me was force me to put my downtime to use by training myself in the Paradox for DOS software, version 3.5. This skill enabled me to escape to UPenn, and later to Wharton, in an attempt to rebrand myself as a *database administrator*, which would have worked, were it not for those meddling kids at Microsoft, who took over the market with Access, while Paradox never translated properly to windows. At UPenn, I did more extensive work with the program, and best of all, grabbed the update to versions 4.0 and 4.5 for $9.95, in my own name (my boss didn't want it), and with that came the Paradox Application Language (PAL), a 4GL database program that enabled me to automate PowerBase, short for ***power rating database***, which kickstarted my financial resurgence, both on and off the basketball court.

My vision after reading ***The Handicapper*** had come to life: I had a working set of power ratings that was guiding me towards profitable betting angles, just as Beyer had destroyed my ROI at the track, save for a few nice winnings streaks in 1993 while I was seeing if continuing the figures was worth it (it wasn't). By contrast, what I called ***speed figures for sports*** offered extreme potential wealth, with a move to Nevada looming increasingly large, as that was the only place to bet legally. I resisted this urge, mostly due to the weather, and the realization that a losing season would leave me stranded in the desert, so I stayed put. Notable is that this opportunity was a direct result of my "low-level" employment.

Two:
Loser Whistleblower Who Lives With Mom

In late 1993, after things didn't work out with UPenn (we have a difference of opinion regarding why), I walked out of Anderson Consulting (now Accenture), then a division of the "legendary" Arthur Anderson and Company, declaring ***I don't take money from Satan*** as my parting shot. Anderson was paying and treating me better than any previous employer, yet they were a microcosm of everything wrong with this country:

- After one employment agency passed me over for a database management assignment at Anderson, another called and sent me, despite the position ***requiring*** a degree. At the interview, I used PowerBase – my adaptation of the Elo rating system from chess to basketball pointspreads – as a sample of my database work, and was hired on the spot at $11.00 an hour.

- For the next eight weeks, I was treated like gold, especially since I'd given the Phillies as my pick to win the National League pennant, which they did, and because I more than tripled my quota of entering 105 fourteen-field records a day from three different source documents, on my first day, relegating the three CPAs on the project to proofreading my work, which was 99.5 percent accurate, thanks to my having to enter a hundred-plus games every Saturday, where mistakes can result in Central Connecticut State being ranked #1.

- The most common question by far regarding PowerBase was always where their ***alma mater*** was ranked. Unlike the quasi-exile of the track, sports betting was mainstream, schedule for working people who could call their bookies before dinner or lunch, and watch the games on evenings and weekends at home, or in packed bars. For the most part, however, I would just call the free scorephones at the end of the night, jot the scores down on my output sheet, then enter them into the program, while for games off the board, I trained my VCR on the ***Headline News Ticker***. Thankfully, this information moved online by 1996, before which I had to make two all-day trips to the library to plug the holes in the data via microfiche copies of newspapers from the past year.

- The project for which I was hired came from a law firm I had quit a month earlier, on the day shift in their word processing center, where I should have worked third shift instead, but by then it was too late. For ten dollars an hour, I could have performed most of the same work that was being billed at a much higher rate, with multiple staff. I calculated that Anderson was making ***$9.00+*** for every dollar they were paying me, which explained why I was allowed to clock out once I finished 350 records, took two-hour lunches paid for by the bosses, and even got rides home.

- I almost became the first nondegreed employee put on staff, but they let me know they were concerned that doing so might set a bad precedent, i.e., eliminate their ability to use the lack of a degree as a reason not to hire someone else, which to me spoke for itself regarding diversity. Of course, ***now*** employers are patting themselves on the back for eliminating degree requirements, but unless they have a time machine set to return me to 1986, it's a little late for me. This, gender bias, and rejection of the merit system combined to cost me six figures or more in lost income, while those who inflicted it looked down on me as inferior, noting my living arrangements.

- When I finally left Anderson in early December, I envisioned America being bankrupted by the bloat and inefficiency I had personally witnessed, with the ***B2B*** sector an exponential amplification of everything wrong with our country. I figured it would take ten or fifteen years for the system to collapse, but had no interest in working "within the system" as it, and its people, were rotten to the core. Lack of diversity (to put it mildly; it was much more blatant) was an issue, but so was my not wanting to spend all day with people I viewed as banal or evil (is there a difference?). From there, I rejected anyone, friend or lover, who got their paychecks from corporate America, instead hanging out with artists, dancers, first responders, and people who were still relatively pure, including college-age women who had yet to be tested by the workforce.

A few days after Anderson, I was hired and then fired from a PAL assignment, due to lack of advanced programming skills. That the firm had two secretarial positions for which I was overqualified, but which paid well, was ignored, as I was sent packing. The financial hit I continued to take was bad enough, but the lack of *meritocracy* scared me, as did discovering just how sick humanity was. In 1991, when I was still minding my business, I noticed teenage girls in catholic school uniforms walking around Center City, thinking it was odd that school ran so late, only to learn that they were coming from law offices who hired only from all-girl schools, and who then required *law office experience* as a barrier to minority women or men, all of which made *#metoo* problems obvious, but my complaints fell on deaf or hostile ears; *don't snitch* is a thing for a reason.

In 1992, I encountered a former female neighbor, now a white-collar professional, who responded to my greeting in a loud, exasperated voice, on the middle of Walnut Street with:

"Aren't you the GUY WHO LIVES WITH HIS <u>MOTHER</u>??"

The woman who slept under the blanket of security I provided at the concierge desk, which my mother managed, was at the time engaged to her now-husband, a highly successful attorney who had also gone to a SUNY school around the same time as me. She was not the first or only UPenn grad student to thumb her nose at me in favor of a wealthy doctor or lawyer, in some cases citing religious reasons for her social-climbing. For *intellectual dishonesty*, nothing comes close to our denial how *transactional* "love" and even "friendship" are (I think of people as *allies* rather than friends, and that's perfectly fine), and it was refreshing for her to actually verbalize her thoughts. I did ponder how proud her husband was to be the man she bragged about, or how she would treat him if he weren't rich.

The Winter Of Twenty-Seven

Seventeen ice storms, my forty-two pound weight loss, coding PowerBase, and writing my first, failed book about said weight loss and its impact on my SMV defined the winter of 1993-94, spent mostly holed up in my apartment, or working the front desk, when I wasn't walking two miles in freezing weather to Market West for my high-intensity workouts. This was the last stop on my whistleblower tour, when I was escorted out of Independence Blue Cross by a very large, muscular, polite security guard, and then informed by Kelly Services that this *Kelly Girl* was no longer on their roster. Preceding this was a snitch-out from the temp I was replacing, and who I figured had no reason to run to the teacher, particularly since he had imposed himself on me by inviting himself to lunch.

The temp, who was fleeing a drunk-driving conviction by working in another state, apparently couldn't stand my speech about why I quit a job where I wouldn't have been hired were I African-American. Defeated, I returned to the desk, PowerBase, the track (sporadically, in search of a new edge), and…*the internet*, which was finally going mainstream. I was tipped off to this new trend by research into the literary marketplace for my weight-loss book, by asking the clerk at *Borders* how many copies of various books had been sold in the previous year. The results were eye-opening:

The clerk who looked up these numbers then mentioned a book that was "taking over the world."

325 *Navigating The Internet*

The weight-loss numbers were encouraging, but the internet book piqued my curiosity, prompting me to subscribe to Prodigy, which required users to buy software and then pay a monthly premium for a service with an antiquated interface that couldn't even keep multiple windows up simultaneously. *PC Link* had just changed its name to *America Online,* a Windows-based service which blew away Prodigy, whose software was free, and which came with an immediate $50.00 credit to cover its $2.95 hourly fee, well worth it given its ubiquitous global reach. Soon after this, a coffeehouse friend of mine from 1991 showed up with a pile of cash, talking about how he was getting rich in *website design*, so I began checking it out. Unfortunately, one needed advanced coding skills and faster PCs than the one paid for by PowerBase to make a website, but it offered a glimpse of the future. Immediately, I saw the distribution potential for the ratings and picks.

The new computer from Boards put Mom and I back in business, this time with paid-off equipment and no expensive maintenance contracts (our *Xerox 6085* system cost several hundred a month to service, and was rendered obsolete in 1988 by the Mac, and UPenn's change to allowing 300 dpi printouts for its resume books). The addition of a 4L printer (bought a few months before the 600-dpi 4P) made us once again a full-service business, for a fraction of what we laid out for the 6085 and its printer, and with no maintenance contract.

In yet another example of just how sick a sociopath Sol was, in 1992, when Mom had a ninety-page job on a 5.5" disk but had to give the client a 3.5" disk, I had to retype the job at another computer, for work. I asked for permission to come in on Saturday and do this, but was denied, an order I disobeyed, sneaking in at dawn to finish before noon, when I *knew* he'd be coming in to check; perhaps he was testing me. A year earlier, a former chess patron refused to use his credit-card to secure a Mac rental for a $3,000.00 job, but someone else came through; I terminated the friendship immediately. We are told to let go of things like this, but how many times is Charlie Brown supposed to try to kick the football before he can tell Lucy to *f**k off?*

Emo types warn us that we have *issues* if we don't turn ourselves into punching bags, usually because they want something from us and don't like our safeguards roadblocking them. Reach my age and lack of status and you'll quickly find no one cares if you hate the world or not, other than to discredit you by claiming you are that bitter, whining loser, in my case living with Mom at age twenty-seven, when all I had to do was not snitch, and my life would have been fine. Thanks to the UPenn grad student's verbal abuse, particularly since she married a man who wouldn't hire me as his secretary, and who may very well have cheated on her with the women he did hire, I advised men not to date *office whores,* as they were unfit for motherhood or marriage.

Men who ignored my warnings to avoid participants in my oppression now comprise much of the *#mgtow* movement, having lost their life savings and any hope of a future, or retirement, to having chosen the wrong woman for marriage, a pitfall I consciously avoided through the sound investment of my time. I may not have had a 401(k), or Roth IRA (which I am now opposed to as it is tax avoidance), but I had plenty of ways to make money even into old age, and more than enough to keep me busy, as the last nine years of my life have shown, just as those who sacrificed their youth for money they almost certainly won't keep until they need it, unless they die first, are staggering to the wire in life, while my *time portfolio* ensures I am never bored. Make no mistake, I am clearly dying, but will remain productive until my last healthy breath, and I have already kept occupied while on borrowed time.

PonytailDude

Continued investment in my time portfolio paid off big in 1994. After my career "ended" at Kelly, I found new life at a securities class-action firm, of the kind started by an old family friend in the 1950s, whose name often turned up on our pleadings. This was paper-pushing law, and very profitable: anytime a stock drops, investor lawsuits would follow, get certified as a class, and the lawyers would get most of the settlement, with some crumbs passed on to the investors. I lasted six weeks there as I was stuck underneath a female (who later became an attorney) that had been hired straight out of high school, had been there six years, and was adored. I was viewed as highly competent, but would never be more than a second fiddle. I did suggest to their African-American receptionist that she try UPenn, for the same reasons I had left, and I did see her smiling at me on Locust Walk on a weekday afternoon about a year later, where she was probably earning double what the law firm paid her, with massive benefits.

The most profound impact the law firm job in the eight weeks or so I was there had on my career occurred after work one evening, when I ducked into a coffeehouse on Twentieth, near Locust, where PonytailDude (see *Bettor Off Single*) was studying chess, which was rare for the venue. I struck up a conversation, and wound up giving him a brutal, three-hour lesson, which he endured without complaint, later thanking me for showing him how to beat the alpha geeks at *The Last Drop* (Thirteenth and Pine), at the time the city's most popular cafe, but one where the women dismissed the "chess guys" as geeks, though we were very popular among the men they wanted.

PonytailDude and I would continue trading chess and PUA knowledge, much as I had done with TrustFundDude in 1991, this time with me in nearly perfect shape from the winter. My game hit the stratosphere, kicking off a three-year period I still can't believe, and wouldn't expect my readers to believe, ending in 1996, when I was using one submissive's AOL account at $2.95 an hour to pick up other women. After the law firm, I placed an ad in the *situations wanted* section of the *Legal Intelligencer,* landing a part-time, $9.00/hour gig for a female solo practitioner building her practice after not making partner at a big firm, the other side of the gender-bias coin. We clicked, a bit too well, as we also dated six times (not really *#metoo* as I was a freelancer).

At the end of 1994, I quit my real-life answer to *The Good Fight*, mostly because the internet was calling; PowerBase was attracting serious interest on the Prodigy and AOL boards, thanks to Banned posting my picks for a 34-17 record that made money for several people. The final tally was seven years of temporary and permanent employment, mostly at around $10.00 an hour, less for the non-overtime hours at the desk, but the dividends continue to this day:

- A year or two in various law offices, teaching me how to litigate and how to defend myself in court, as well as filing my own bankruptcy in 1998.

- Two years as a medical secretary, giving me invaluable knowledge of and contacts within the healthcare industry.

- A year with a CPA firm, which taught me how to do my own accounting, and to avoid hiring accountants and lawyers, who will take my business plan and sell it as a consulting product to wealthier clients who can crush me with distribution and infrastructure.

- Knowledge and a copy of Paradox 4.5 for DOS, which I use to this day for my betting and trading bots, and without which I would be lost as a handicapper or daytrader. In retirement, this offers not only jackpot and profit potential, but a ***cost-free hobby*** that yields hours of enjoyment and enhancement for my sports betting experience.

- ***Free time***, and time on the desk job, which allowed me to train fulltime at chess, delve fulltime into handicapping, and even allow me to do freelance work while working the front desk (best of both worlds), as well as to be around whenever a woman I wanted was available, rather than being stuck in an office and unable to deploy the six-figure income which attracted her. All in all, I was quite content, even if my retirement would suck.

America Goes Online

In 1995, the internet was completely up for grabs, with seemingly infinite potential for generating wealth. That potential still exists, but has been commandeered by ***tolltakers*** on the information superhighway who use their market dominance and censorship power to stifle anyone who points out that their existence is unnecessary at best, and illegal at worst. The seeds for the toxic internet you see now were planted in the mid-1990s, mostly to prevent people like me from becoming wealthy, while painting me as a ***bitter, whining loser who lives with his mother and blames others for his failures in life.*** Like the school bullies I avoided by cutting a hundred twenty days a year, I felt no obligation to engage my abusers, and felt pity for those who did, on the mistaken belief they would never be targeted. "Next time it might happen to someone you care about" was a popular refrain.

How sexy was ***Tanya?*** That's SHBWitchy from ***Bettor Off Single***, and I'm not sure I ever got her last name. She was twenty when we met over AOL in the ***Spring of Twenty-Eight.*** I taught her hypnosis (something I rarely write about, due to intellectual dishonesty and public ignorance), and was ready to fly to Oregon to meet and probably marry her, since she was determined to find a husband, and equally determined to make sure it was me. Instead, Nick Anderson missed four free throws in Game One of the NBA Finals against the Rockets, after leading by twenty just before the half. With only $1,400.00 to make the trip, I had risked $300.00 to win what I needed to cover the full trip, but when this failed, I was left with $1,100.00 in cash, the proceeds of typing two books, historical texts by African-American scholar Merzie Wilson, a far more enlightening and rewarding experience than big-firm consulting. When I asked why she hired a white guy, she said she heard I was the best.

<u>**Sexxretary**</u>

With all day and night to kill online, I engaged in one of the first *catfish* expeditions, with the above screen name. My *100 wpm typing* positioned me to appear authentic to the office predators, who fell hook, line, and sinker, at times offering legitimate jobs in the mid-to-high five figures. The "highlight reel" was quite disgusting:

- A lawyer from Manhattan who made clear that sex was a job requirement, and who even gave me the name of a female attorney at the EEOC as he laughed off my reveal, as if *stealing* that money from my pocket, or the pockets of any woman not sufficiently attractive or compromised. Having already had a complaint against Temple University ignored back in 1991, I saw no point in filing another. In 1995, I chided Bill Cosby for telling minorities not to "whine" about discrimination, calling him human excrement; it seems I was early.

- A cable executive who offered *$110,000.00 a year* for an executive assistant/hooker, verified.

- Countless men who asked if I took *D**Ktation*, but these were not serious offers.

What would become clear to the world through *#metoo* was well known back in the *Lewinsky* era, where Monica made $32,000.00 a year in the White House, and turned down many $50,000.00+ "hush money" jobs in Manhattan after outing Clinton. Somehow, when I pointed out that men were generally not considered for any job where sexual harassment was claimed, no one cared, nor did anyone care that I had taken a stand against racism by quitting a job over lack of diversity. It became clear very quickly that most either were not aware of how bad sexual harassment was, or if they did, they participated if male, or profited if female. The mere mention of what we now openly acknowledge, like *#prettyprivilege*, sent "office whores" and horny bosses alike into fits of intellectually dishonest rage.

Of my dual existence, the half that did not have to interact with others (chess, PowerBase, writing, freelancing, coding) ran like clockwork, while anything requiring others (employment, friendships, or relationships with women who worked in offices) was stopped dead in its tracks. Instead of spending my prime years in Manhattan, running a third-shift word processing department at a law firm, making $75,000.00 a year, and owning a quarter-million dollar co-op which would now be worth a few million. Unlike my time portfolio, my financial trajectory was stalled, with no real hope other than a jackpot.

Without question, I would never have developed my outside interests much at all had I spent all my time at a job building my nest egg. Each lost experience can radically alter enjoyment later in life: while Mr. Shaibel was not a very strong player, he found fulfillment in coaching Beth Harmon, but *Benny Watts* is the type of player I wanted to be in my old age: still strong, and able to influence the higher levels of the game, as I did when I defeated Tariq Yue. In theory, it's easier to be able to fund your passions, and to bet only money you can afford to lose, yet it is **_not_** being funded, and **_not_** able to afford losses that will sharpen you in the long run. It doesn't have to be life or death, more like steak or Ramen noodles, depending on whether or not you win. After a big win, Mom and I always splurged around $40.00 on the *obligatory celebratory Chinese food dinner*, with my favorite dish, Fillet Steak.

Shrinkage And IUJohn

The vast reaches of the internet, which stretched IRL (in real life), had me more optimistic about he future than at any point since 1991, though I had never really lost hope. ***Living with Mom*** allowed me to devote time to those "waste of life" pursuits which now comprise my retirement time portfolio. Best of all was not having to reveal my situation to anyone, including women, until Mom's ignorance literally put a ***doxing*** target on my back, when she demanded we register our first website in her name. The egalitarian internet, if it ever existed, was being clamped down upon by commercial interests and censorship, and then Section 230 giving immunity for defamation, effectively creating an open season which sociopaths like Kenneth "Shrink" Weitzner were able to exploit.

In 1995, I held a contest on the AOL sports betting message board, where a handicapper known only as IUJohn and I dueled to the wire, each picking around 65 percent winners for the NCAA basketball conference season. We were patting ourselves on the back in the private ***PowerChat,*** when a square stopped by to let us know we were ***12-0*** whenever we agreed on a game, and offered to send us money, which we declined. I wasn't worried, since these weren't the Beyer figures, and my edge wasn't going anywhere, or so I thought. On the downside, basketball was only four months a year, and only two of those (January-February) were reliably profitable, though the NFL came through for me most years.

This was not simple handicapping but further compounding of my interest as I continued to build on Dad's training, and what I had learned from ***The Handicapper***, mainly that power ratings could in fact beat the bookie, indicating my efforts would not be wasted, and they were not. I had found my replacement for the track, which was also beginning to return to profitability. I was preparing PowerBase for national distribution, with $10,000.00+ in advertising to ***Athlon's*** and ***Street & Smith's*** yearbooks, the latter part of the ***Condé Nast*** family of publications designed to break even while generating a lucrative mailing list. Rather than just cash in immediately on AOL, I used the same ***patience and discipline*** which cost me a small fortune at the track in 1986, rather than just cashing in.

As it turned out, I seriously underestimated my competition on two fronts: Shrink had connections to a top syndicate, for which he moved money, so the ***scamdicapper*** label didn't apply, but he also had insider connections at AOL and with the feds, for whom he was an informant. Apparently, he saw me as a threat long before I realized who he was, as his 24-17 record in the contest (a solid 58.5 percent) did not stand out against me or IUJohn, but he was laying in wait for baseball season, when everyone but him would be on the sidelines preparing for the NFL.

With the ad set to drop in September, 1996, my winnings, and stable income from the desk and freelancing, I was well-positioned to finally make some progress. For most of 1995-96, I enjoyed life, spending most of my time with the online and offline ***harems*** I had built, not really aware of how abnormal my results with women had become. Finally, the 1996 NFL season approached, with me giving out selections to market PowerBase; Shrink was not pleased.

VegasDude

Another fortune slipped through my fingers in 1995, when I refused to swallow my ego and just bet on picks from VegasDude, one of my few paying PowerBase clients, who sent me $250.00 for the season's ratings without batting an eye. He envisioned me as a protégé of sorts, and we'd pass time during the day exchanging ideas and picks, with his almost never losing, including one involving Green Bay -4.5 and under-44, which they won 24-19, for an example of how *precise* he was. Through this man, I was connected to the syndicates, as well as through a friend at a bookie's in New York, but I wanted not just to win, but to win with ***PowerBase***. Had I simply pumped gas, saved my money and wagered on the syndicate picks I was getting, I'd have become wealthy. Instead, I wound up in Shrink's crosshairs for having the temerity to compete on his digital "turf."

When I wasn't chatting with VegasDude, Shrink and I would chat for up to a few hours a day while waiting for lines, often commenting on the message board. This is when he revealed his connection to the syndicates, for whom he moved millions of dollars a year, making a good living for himself, apparently while collecting disability payments. He was not an actual psychiatrist, but had taken the medical boards before giving up on that career. I learned how volatile he was when he threatened to ***kill*** me after I joked about sleeping with his wife if he lost a big bet, and not in a joking manner. After that, I kept my distance, but it was too late. He also knew I lived with Mom because we were on the phone so much, and didn't hesitate to use that to discredit me, warning the audience that I couldn't be much of a handicapper if I didn't have my own place.

I could have survived Shrink's disparagement if he hadn't won with his syndicate picks, but even then he still had connections inside AOL, which he used to get my account nuked, taking my advertising campaign with it, as the e-mail contact was on this account. Had I gone into business with him, I'd have cashed in, but I wanted nothing to do with the syndicates and potential money-laundering issues, the same reason I did not partner up with VegasDude, instead just sharing my ratings in exchange for the syndicate picks that I did not use. Sharp sports bettors tend to gravitate towards each other, since combining their knowledge increases the winning percentage and ROI. PowerBase was my entry into this culture, beginning in 1993, when I started betting with New York offices.

Unfortunately, between the winning picks winning over the audience, and his ability to nuke my account, my attempt to commercialize PowerBase was a complete failure: the program, which has hit 61.8 percent the past four years in the NFL, ***sold not a single copy*** to an audience that cries out for winning picks and methods, only to dismiss anyone who claims to have them as a con artist or know-it-all. Despite my living with Mom to cut costs and to enable riskier bets that might lead to a breakthrough, I was dismissed as a ***loser in Mom's basement,*** even though we had no basement, and I was paying half the bills while a partner in the new family word processing service, for which I had supplied paid-off equipment.

Shrink's intellectual dishonesty foreshadowed what everyone now experiences on the postmodern internet, with doxing, defamation, harassment, disinformation, censorship, shadowbanning, false advertising, and fraud all thrive, mostly thanks to Section 230 of the Communications Decency Act of 1996, which immunized internet companies and search engines from liability for third-party content or any claims that they were a publisher (or distributor) of online libel, allowing them to remain unscathed for allowing Shrink to destroy my reputation and business, along with those of anyone else he perceived as a threat.

In 1997, I was a financial ***dead man walking***, awaiting the final shoe to drop with a creditor lawsuit that would sink me into bankruptcy. Shrink even tried to do business with me, because he wanted access to my horse racing audience, which had become substantial, thanks to the ***United Free***

Handicappers newsletter that did not compete with Shrink directly, but this did not stop his paranoia, which was on full display the day after the 1997 NBA Finals, when my phone rang, followed by numerous threats of federal prosecution from a bogus FBI agent on three-way calling, apparently over some antisemitic postings on his website. I told him the "agent" could use internet records to verify that it wasn't me.

Millionaires' Lounge

The infamous AOL chat was noted for its authenticity and presence of multiple confirmed millionaires, who in turn attracted large numbers of exceptionally hot, *looks-verified* golddiggers, back in the day when *catfishing* was presumed. The chat showed that women cared not at all about merit, right and wrong, or how the wealthy men in their lives got their money, which they were able to control very easily, like the *$1 million* in venture capital one arranged for me, then cancelled when I noted why she had such influence with my wannabe investor for a "stock market website" that could easily have become dominant with the right backing. Not long after this, a death threat from the investor came: *"you'll never know what hit you,"* playing to the stereotype of the omnipotent, sociopathic rich. *"At least the cops will know where to look,"* I replied.

With no path to solvency, I filed for Chapter 7 bankruptcy in 1998, without an attorney, giving "employment discrimination" as the official cause at the Meeting of Creditors, where I was the only one in attendance. My case was discharged in April, giving me a fresh start. I had learned as a paralegal that bankruptcy was a huge plus to lenders, because it meant I had no debt, couldn't file again for six more years, and that clearing the decks meant I was expecting my income to spike and to pay my bills going forward, which I was. Meanwhile, Shrink was betraying everyone who stayed on board past his winning streak, when he went from charging $400.00 a month to giving away his picks, while taking from the sportsbooks up to 50 percent of money lost by those he referred. He got paid on the way up and down for many who ignored me at his urging, along with my warning that he couldn't be trusted.

Shrink and his wife, who embraced his behavior since she profited from it, committed suicide in 2010, after he lost $700,000.00 in the NCAA tournament, apparently thanks to his syndicate buddies giving him the wrong side of games. Fourteen years later, I'm still standing, with sports betting now legal and mainstream in a way that Shrink did not live long enough to see; he'd have loved it. I may not have broken the bank the way he did, but I also avoided the slugs and the swamp which eventually claimed his life, though by then the audience that helped him steal unearned millions from people like me no longer cared.

The Bankrupt Pickup Artist

That someone with my education and skills would ever have to file a Chapter 7 Bankruptcy, as I did in April, 1998, is nothing short of an *atrocity*, but this was not the world's concern, since the *99 percent* was cruising along just fine, even thriving during the dotcom bubble. Millions of people could have fixed this overnight, yet once I was tagged as a whistleblower, in addition to being a strong minority in my job category, people were either too scared to speak up or help, or they were on the other side, harassing women or enabling those who do. What was truly maddening was how, when I pointed out that a world that allowed this to happen to me was full of people to avoid, I was attacked again as the *bitter, whining loser who lived with Mom*, even though it was their conduct which made that necessary.

Watching women summarily reject men for this reason, even if some did not, showed them to be morally bankrupt, and likely to wind up with men just like them, as I noted in my PUA work.

My atrocious financial condition belied a life I had come to enjoy a great deal, outside of the intensifying harassment I was receiving from many corners of the internet:

- ♦ A group of hypnotists who didn't like my article entitled ***High School Stage Hypnotists RAPE CHILDREN*** (they do), and took it upon themselves to dox, defame, and harass me, including hiring a private investigator who let me know he "got close" to me near my home, and to make repeated death threats against me, and even Mom.

- ♦ A pair of gymnastics groupies, one of whom is now a famous Hollywood producer, took it upon themselves to "defend" elite gymnasts against my claims of rampant child abuse in the sport. Their narrative was that I was a ***pedophile*** who used fabricated abuse allegations to inject myself into the sport and the lives of its gymnasts, stereotyping me as that ***creepy loser who lives with Mom***, all the while one of the coaches and ringleaders was covering up for sexual abuse at her gym, as she revealed in a newspaper article years later. Even the FBI ignored my warnings, which may have enabled Larry Nassar's abuse, though I was focused on physical abuse documented in works like ***Little Girls in Pretty Boxes.*** Around this time (1998), a top gymnast ran away, confirming my story, but the search-engine damage had been done.

- ♦ The gymnastics groupies impersonated my mother on a USENET post to a sex newsgroup that included our address and phone number, with an invitation to strange men to visit or call. Four called, I answered, and they hung up. When that didn't silence me, they built a doxing website to which they'd link in response to my USENET posts, and even wrote a sick essay about raping and murdering the Olympic gymnasts, to which they signed my name, ***from an ISP I have never used,*** making it impossible for me to have been the author. Despite this, Google did not remove all of the posting (section 230), which is still linked to by others to this day, causing ongoing harm to my reputation, and acting out from wannabe internet vigilantes, though this has subsided over time.

The burgeoning ***pickup artist (PUA) community*** latched on to the lies told to discredit me in other USENET groups, specifically alt.romance, soc.singles, alt.hypnosis, and rec.gambling.sports, and alt.sport.gymnastics, creating an unholy alliance of gymnasts and PUAs which were clear red flags that went unnoticed by a public that was rewarding this hate marketing with their business, and in the process harming themselves by relying on misinformation, like the losers Shrink intentionally gave out in order to snag affiliate commissions based on his "sheet's" losses to the house. A medium that was supposed to make truth impossible to suppress had accomplished the opposite, as it came to be dominated by commercial interests, either AOL's in its proprietary approach to commerce (even e-mailing PowerBase updates to an opt-in list violated their TOS), which ultimately gave way to social media censorship, all desired by the public, despite its protestations, as it abandoned USENET.

<u>WTF!? You're Just Telling Lame Stories</u>

If you are saying something like this, you are the problem:

> ***Hey man I know you had a rough life and have to talk about it nonstop but man GET OVER IT and STOP WASTING MY TIME now can SOMEONE on here tell me how to seduce these bitches my ex-wife just cleaned me in court!! p.s. u <u>live with UR MOM</u> no woman wants that!! p.p.s. u act like every boss is a rapist and every secretary a whore maybe UR ATTITUDE is why u didn't get hired!!***

Negative outcomes have negative causes, often very complex, and which will often challenge one's world view. As one ASF regular put it, if we knew what was wrong with our "game" we'd fix it or realize we couldn't, but we don't, which is why we keep repeating our mistakes with no clue as to why they occur. In the above case, laziness, entitlement, cynicism, and a desire for social advancement through bullying and verbal aggression give rise to the poor results with women, while also causing him to ignore or dismiss long-winded, complex explanations. This mindset also has men like this dismissing PowerBase because of men like Shrink, who ultimately con him out of his money, while appealing to his base instincts by noting that a ***loser who lives with his Mommy*** couldn't possibly be winning, while being impressed by Shrink's wealth, even as he fed that wealth to him thanks to intellectual dishonesty, of the same kind that misleads people into sacrificing their youth for a nest egg.

Loudmouthed bullies are a serious problem, but even more serious is the audience of ***useful idiots*** who stand down while they hijack center stage in a pathetic attempt to get noticed. At college, someone who knew Kate once made a power play at my expense, by rising from his table and declaring that "everyone" didn't like me, only tolerating me because that I smoked weed with them, which I already knew, but since I had a roommate who didn't allow me to smoke in the room (which was against the rules of course), I had no alternatives. I didn't strike back, just looking at him and his friends, and continuing, which impressed Kate no end (she later praised me in a bar for keeping my cool).

Examples like the above occur repeatedly on the internet, and when no one calls them out, people like me won't bother, since those who claim to want my knowledge or help don't have my back when attempting to provide it, whether it is sports picks and the Shrink, or love advice and the typical ***entitled snowflake*** trying to blend in with the popular kids (studies show most bullying is an attempt at social advancement). Since the popular kids have excluded me my entire life (I began bowling one afternoon after being ***left out*** of a pickup softball game despite being able to hit home runs at age nine), I gravitated naturally towards individual sports and solitary pastimes, and later jobs or hobbies, that require ***little to no interaction with others***. The list of ***atrocities*** I have endured reflects why: I was not singled out at all, but instead moved through a world that has no room for people like me. Ambushes like this are so common that I expect them, another reason I don't trust strangers or even acquaintances.

If you can't handle complicated explanations, that's not my problem. These are literally my ***last words***, or something close, and they are taking time from my chess training, betting, and daytrading. I'd say I'm doing this for the readers but at the end of the day it is for myself and my legacy, though in the course of serving that aim I provide information I believe to be useful to those who want to understand ***my*** way of life, not theirs. The painstaking details offer a glimpse into just how difficult it is to swim against the tide and emerge from the ***river of shit*** that is intellectual dishonesty. Men are in total crisis with women, sports bettors lose money, and people wind up screwed in retirement with nothing to offer beyond money they no longer have, all because they threw in with the wrong people and believed the wrong ideas, yet they ridicule anyone who has the answers they claim to seek.

My lack of a nest egg kept me driven not just for financial stability, but to become so wealthy that retirement would take care of itself, though even then it usually does not, given the prohibitive cost of healthcare in retirement and the spend-down requirements. While this was a concern, I had become a "dating expert" in 1991 simply to answer a woman's question about my line of work with something other than ***Kelly Girl.*** I also realized that women love talking about sex and relationships, since this attracts men without their having to put out. Though not my original intent, the internet exploded both the market for dating advice, and the level of interaction between author and reader, making this arena the most promising, after sports betting had crashed and burned. It was also a platform for my gender politics, as I had linked employment and romantic outcomes with regard to office work. Hilarity ensued.

The PUA community was born from censorship, itself born from intellectual dishonesty, specifically the narrative that ***women like nice guys***, men were jerks, and the AOL and prodigy boards, which were dominant at the time, devolved into quasi-dating fora where ***simps*** would "defend women," while calling out "misogynist" men like me, who posted unflattering views of the opposite sex, such as women being social-climbers (hypergamy), and how they reward "badboy" behavior. My goal was to market CUPID, my compatibility algorithm, which I had converted into a "love life management database" in Paradox, though it never caught fire. What did catch fire was ***Outfoxing The Foxes*** (1998), an advice book in which CUPID comprised the first four chapters, followed by what I believed the reader should do with the information and ratings. CUPID itself was very simple:

Category	Women	Men
Looks	55%	80
Brains	20	10
Money/Status	20	10
Personality	05	05

For compatibility between specific individuals, the ***partner rating*** was calculated using individual values, rather than the universal ones for the generic, "societal" rating; a sapiosexual is more likely to have something like a 40-40-20 split. Each category was scored on a 1-25 scale, and weighted above. My bodybuilding during the ***Winter of Twenty-Seven*** confirmed this, as it shot up my CUPID rating by almost thirty points, while for women, anatomy really is destiny, as my fashionista hater informed me in 1986 while advising me to avoid the track.

Before I ***looksmaxed,*** sapiosexuals – I called them ***minddiggers*** – were almost my entire dating pool, since even the gorgeous ones put so much emphasis on intellect that to them I had an elite rating, much like any man with money will appeal to golddiggers, while almost every man and many women classify as ***looksdiggers***. What I neglected to account for with this desirability rating was marriage-mindedness. Kate, who I wanted to marry, had a perfect score, but remains single to this day.

Netgirl, Censorship, And USENET

Netgirl was AOL's brand for its dating-advice boards, which competed with Prodigy for market dominance, gradually prevailing as the latter receded from the marketplace. Thanks to PowerBase having me online, I passed a lot of time on Netgirl, posting how women who worked in offices should be avoided because of sexualized hiring, with sexual harassers controlling their work environment, using the story of how one of my ex-bosses continued interviewing women for my first full week on the job, calming my fears of doing poorly by letting me know he just liked having women alone in his office begging him for work. A few years earlier, a temp I worked with told me about a woman who had to ***kiss her boss on the lips*** every morning to remain employed.

What is now taken for granted thanks to *#metoo* had people calling me mentally ill, delusional, and of course a ***bitter, whining loser who lives with his mother***, and therefore should not be taken seriously, effectively ***ad hominem*** on steroids. Nowhere is our intellectual dishonesty on parade more than in the dating-advice arena, and I was smack in the middle of its ground zero, about to move to its new ground zero, USENET, thanks to censorship of "misogyny" on AOL that was costing me my accounts. I was never silenced, as I kept up to four backup accounts to deploy in case one was nuked, but it was very annoying to have to repeatedly change my screen names. AOL was like Studio 54; when it went down in 1996 for nineteen hours, it led the national news, a sign the internet had arrived.

Hate Speech Violates TOS!

The PUA community was spawned by censorship on AOL and Prodigy, which sent the most knowledgeable men to USENET, to join ***Speed Seduction*** creator Ross Jeffries (a/k/a Paul Ross), whose application of ***neurolinguistic programming*** (NLP) to seduction, which Tracy Cabot introduced in ***How To Make A Man Fall In Love With You***, and which I had read about in 1985. The ***alt.seduction.fast*** (ASF) group was created to separate "SS" traffic from the noncommercial discussions in ***alt.romance*** and ***soc.singles***. This was USENET's heyday, in an era where e-mail could take several days (Shrink's power stemmed from AOL's monopoly on instant e-mail within its servers, a must in a time-sensitive industry), whereas newsgroups were global and published in realtime. ASF was controversial given its commercial influence, but the lesser of all evils. Another group, ***alt.seduction.outfoxing***, was created for my work, but my haters crossed over and made that irrelevant, so I returned to ASF.

The battle for an audience worth tens of millions of dollars made ASF and USENET a much higher-stakes environment than meets the eye, just like the AOL sports betting boards were the battleground for competing touts. Social media censorship had yet to clamp down on the free speech on which USENET thrived, but its progenitors took shape, in the form of commercial websites promoted in the "ASF FAQ" document, normally for ***frequently asked questions*** about a newsgroup, but which was hijacked into promoting the group's "main websites," while claiming they were just like USENET, which they were, except for commercialization and censorship, which I considered intellectually dishonest, particularly given that men were altering their love lives based on what they found on ASF.

Since most women reject ***losers who live with their mother***, I became easy prey for disparagement, even if I was having sex with women on my roof, at their place, or even in a center city hotel while I was "visiting" my hometown. Very quickly, the "community," if there ever was one, evolved into what I called the ***Seduction Mafia*** in a lawsuit, and which Ross Jeffries himself called the ***Seduction Syndicate*** in 2010, after he had a falling out with some members of the group. That it was ***my*** techniques that were being co-opted and spread, along with Mystery's, Ross's, and a number of others, was ironic. My "pivot" technique of using a female friend to build a reputation as a ladies' man was met with scorn until its success, which fueled ASF going mainstream, as more and more men were suddenly getting laid. This couldn't last, and I predicted ***game over*** would follow. One of my haters, who called me a pedophile every chance he got, was eventually convicted of possession of child pornography in 2011.

Three:
Resurgence (1999-2002)

While my haters were attempting to destroy my reputation and business online, including the use of several ***death threats***, my time portfolio grew exponentially in the above years, as my PUA books were taking off, my love life was still going strong, PowerBase had found its stride, and thanks to PAP (short for ***price and probability***), I returned to profitability at the racetrack, shortly after releasing ***How To Break Even At The Track*** in 1999, which sold well at $39.95 a copy, for an audience of rebated players who could profit from churning their bankroll, something not available in Pennsylvania, and the other reason I almost moved to Nevada in 1995, as they offered nine percent. The internet was finding its stride as well, particularly the PUA community, even as the dotcom bubble burst and the future seemed bleak. After September 11, 2001, the world changed, but the internet remained in a long-term holding pattern, awaiting its next quantum leap, which came with the advent of social media a few years later.

It is said that we don't know what we have until it's gone, but I definitely knew what I had, and that it would vanish soon enough, particularly in my love life. HBChina (see ***Bettor Off Single***) was an award-winning singer (Chinese MTV) and medical Doctor. I made my move on her in tandem with my racetrack resurgence, after waiting an hour in the cold for the #21 bus on Chestnut Street, for a trip to Garden State Park to put $75.00 on Menifee at 19-1 in the Derby futures, along with some $10.00 backups, including the winner, Charismatic (15-1 in the mutuel field). I saw HBChina in the lobby, asked her for a ride, and offered her wagers on all of my horses, which she could then drive us back to collect, after which I had a date planned.

Menifee missed by a head in the Derby, costing me about $3,000.00 compared to the ***$550.00*** I made on the race. I did cash on Charismatic, putting me in HBChina's car yet again, but instead of a date, we went back to her apartment. She lit up like a Christmas tree when I expressed an interest in hypnosis, but I didn't cash in immediately, instead choosing to toy with my prey, as I had already climbed every PUA mountain and knew she wanted me, effectively outsmarting myself. I had actually been winning since July, 1998, when I published daily selections under the campaign ***Ray Gordon CLOBBERS Saratoga,*** to mock the scamdicappers with outrageous claims that I somehow made real with a $1.20 ROI on all selections, and double my money on best bets, as my PAP power rating method began taking shape and showing extreme promise, prompting ***Break Even***, which was also cross-marketed to my PUA audience. Registering my publishing company so that I could retain income and creative control over my work also led to several editing and manuscript jobs, some over four figures.

The Social-Security Widow's Benefit (Age Sixty)

Retirement planning is about much more than hoarding tax-advantaged money for use later in life. Sometimes ignorance can be costly, as it was for Mom, who turned sixty in 1999 and could have retired, handing the desk manager's job and her transcription clients over to me, which would have boosted my income, while taking the Social Security widow's benefit in May, when she turned sixty. This would have made my own retirement/disability check larger, but instead she continued working, which was also fine, but a lot more effort on her part. I still had no nest egg, as my immediate priorities were overwhelming my cash, which is why I continued to develop PAP, PowerBase, and my internet career, to the extent I could improve my finances without destroying my time portfolio, which I believed was ultimately the best path to retirement security, even if it did not seem that way.

Though not financially stable or secure, I was making more than enough money to survive, with an increasing threat to break the bank on multiple fronts. That *women* did not value this in no way detracted from its value, though the way they judged men like me certainly gaslit other men into following intellectually dishonest paths such as building a nest egg for the healthcare system that will leave them destitute and, worse, *boring* in old age. As I continued to build on my foundation, my life became increasingly *interesting*, with everything I did being done at a much higher level than "checkers in a nursing home." Instead, I was paired against Hikaru Nakamura in a Sunday morning tournament on ICC, while giving dating advice that changed the world, and making high-stakes wagers that offered a genuine chance at wealth, even producing a profitable, PG-13 hypnosis mp3 on the way. Life was fun.

Timing, and other events beyond one's control, play a huge role in retirement wealth. Even during the dotcom bubble, investing in stocks and options was next to impossible, with even "discount" brokers still charging $14.95 a trade, grinding the *velocity of money* to a halt. In the 1980s, commissions were so high that they exceeded the cost of my entire bankroll, which they still did, since I had already rolled up smaller amounts into four figures multiple times, at which point I could have bought some long-term investments, but that's a good way to get trapped if the situation changes; we are intellectually dishonest when we advise against timing the market, since literally every trade attempts this, and can wind up stuck with a loser because liquidating each time a bet doesn't pan out was too expensive. By contrast, I had turned $6.00 into $500.00 in 1983, and $15.00 into thousands in 1986, bet sizes which wouldn't have covered even a single commission back then, but which now are a full bankroll.

Midnight Train To Georgia

In September, 2000, I briefly hit bottom, after being physically threatened by a restaurant owner who had a *WaiTRESS Wanted* sign in his front window, after I called him out for gender discrimination. I'm not sure how he would have dealt with the police after threatening me, but I decided I had enough and made and applied to the Social Security Administration for disability benefits (SSDI), given that I couldn't find work, and some were using my *attitude* as a pretext, plus I had been diagnosed as bipolar after my suicide attempt, though I was not on medication and had no criminal record. I wound up missing the appointment thanks to Earl "Brother" Jones, former DA of Albany, Georgia, and his daughter, Stefanie, who was in very poor health, but recruited me to begin work on October 1, 2000, at a salary of $500.00 a week (minus the cost of my rented furniture), and a *signing bonus* of $2,500.00, most of which I spent during my four-week *staycation* leading up. I felt like a true alpha male!

- I reconnected with HBChina, finally moving in for the kill at dawn, after spending the night talking in her living room, where she called me to help with an alleged assignment she couldn't explain to me, a likely pretext for a hookup. I took her up to the roof, intending to hypnotize her as the sun rose, and she followed my lead eagerly. Unfortunately, a *homeless couple* was on the roof, destroying a year of progress, after which the spell was broken, and the mood spoiled. I point this out primarily because *living with Mom* was a plus to her, and she didn't care about my financial planning for retirement, yet many men squander their youth at work without regard to how they would attract a woman like HBChina, with whom most men would never have a chance.

- I picked up a stripper at *Wizzard's*, who refused my money, gave me her number, which I called, then played it cool for a week before calling her back, when her number was changed. In Albany, someone found me on ASF and e-mailed me for advice, claiming she was his girlfriend (not sure it wasn't her), which meant he was asking for help with the stripper he swiped from me! I gave the advice, then asked why she changed her number.

- In Albany, I was one of the highest-earning nondegreed men, better educated, and a very good catch to a number of young ladies looking to escape to bigger cities. My love life took off almost immediately. One morning, I was on the bus with a woman who got off a stop before mine, only to find a message on my desk from her with her number. She lived near me so we were always crossing paths. The bars were also packed with singles.

- As it turned out, a $3,000.00 transcription job turned up just after I left Philadelphia, and my horrific 4-17 start to the NFL, just as I was marketing PowerBase via ***The Revolution Guide To Sports Betting***, reversed into a season-long winning streak that continued to the end of basketball. An 8-0 run in the playoffs, and futures and moneyline bets on the Ravens, had me picking up a second paycheck from my bookie, who would move the lines off my relatively small bets, which is why I was never ***Banned4Life***. Fast-forward to today when winning bettors are used as marketing and it would take tens of millions of dollars to get banned, though they will restrict limits, but with today's menu that is hardly an impediment. Like horse racing, Daily Fantasy (DFS) is parimutuel.

- On February 1, 2001, I was sent packing, as the firm downsized. Within a few years, Brother and Stefanie, as well as their other paralegal, had died, dissolving the firm, which hired me after their only two staff for six years quit on the same day. I had made a career out of turning chaos into an opportunity to rebuild their office, and went to town, creating templates in Word that they used until the end. I had finally found that well-paying office job, but had to go to the deep south to do it. I also saw the 2000 election from a different viewpoint than up north, while also missing the subway series in New York, during the John Rocker controversy. Interesting times!

- On my way to the airport in Atlanta, I scrambled to find a ***Kinko's*** to use their computer to place my basketball bets, winning $75.00 when a 5½-point favorite won by six in overtime. The next evening, I won $385.00 at the Meadowlands off an exacta box picked from the tote board (they were well below their morning line), which seemed to be much more accurate than handicapping.

- Because I was earning money, and hadn't sought credit, my credit score took off, and I wound up with eight cards shortly after bankruptcy, putting me in a position where I might have to file again in 2004, but I was living in the present, with no intention of failing, which of course was possible.

Upon my return to Philadelphia, I was determined to level the playing field, and filed an EEOC complaint against UPenn. I also filed against a temp agency which didn't use me, settling the case for $1,000.00 by refuting what I considered intellectual dishonesty:

> ***THEM:*** "He was poorly dressed, did not make a good impression, and had a poor attitude," said the placement counselor who interviewed me.

> ***ME:*** "I had three interviews with temp agencies that day. Immediately after this interview, I had another, and with the same clothes, and attitude, I was hired immediately."

Proving discrimination is much easier than getting the courts to care about it, so I took the money. While some have called me litigious, I was merely defending my rights, using paralegal skills I had deliberately acquired as part of my "slacker" employment, in a way anyone else would have if they had done the same. Being denied work, or defamed online by business rivals, creates genuine damage, and people who don't want to be sued shouldn't give people reasons to sue them. Recent decisions abolishing affirmative-action have proven me right, but long after they are of any use to me. Nature will usually fix injustice rather than any individual, as also occurred with *#metoo*. Activism and whistleblowing are often a futile, premature, and redundant sacrifice.

The temp assignment, for a trade publication whose primary income was from ***advertorials*** (another form of intellectual dishonesty to some), was about as boring, mundane, and mindless as a job could be, but it was a bare-bones $10.00 an hour, four days a week, enough to pay my bills while preserving an extra day for my time portfolio. It also allowed me to remain solvent while fighting UPenn, in the hope of abolishing affirmative action, which would open up tens of thousands of jobs to me, in a favorable legal climate. This made sense, because the status quo ensured that my retirement money would not be coming from the scraps left over after the women took all the best jobs. My freelance income, winnings, and now book royalties served only to plug the income hole, when they should have been augmenting a nice paycheck.

Focusing on what for most are hobbies rather than a retirement plan was logical, continuously building on a solid foundation to reach very high levels in multiple areas. That too would change when, in 2002, an area psychologist and subcontractor for DHS hired me to transcribe a dozen or so reports each week, at a rate of $4.00 a single-spaced page. This worked out to a very steady $200.00+ a week, for work which took me eight to ten hours, but which I never finished early, lest my client question my rate. My weekends became a mix of horse racing and transcription, and on a side note regarding intellectual dishonesty, when my footpedal broke, I found that a "listen and repeat" technique was quicker and more accurate, saving a lot of money on equipment.

The internet has only amplified people's obsession with finances and retirement, as evidenced by the ***FIRE*** movement, and its counterpart that advises us to maximize our twenties, as I did. Jettisoning this concern allowed me to focus on my time portfolio much more than most, and it now pays the dividends I had expected much earlier. By late 2002, I was well on the way to where I wanted to be, perhaps even becoming wealthy enough to retire much earlier than one would expect of someone without a nest egg at thirty-five. As I aged, women faded into the background, since PUA is a young man's game, and this made life much more uncomplicated and inexpensive, while my experience with both my occupations and avocations brought more and more opportunity and enjoyment.

While I was in a holding pattern, and never stopped making progress towards the retirement I now enjoy, there were many bumps along the way, yet they never derailed me, only altering the trajectory a few times.

Four:
The Law Office (2002-2009)

Mom used to remark that *the Law Office is open* whenever I worked on litigation of my various cases involving UPenn, internet rivals, or others. Most of the cases wound up dismissed, but the final two yielded a win and a settlement, before I *delitigated* in 2009. This was also a very profitable period for betting, with PAP and PowerBase stronger and more profitable than ever. I reverted to my childhood spending habits from the UES, no longer concerned about money, spending it on everything from expensive meals out, to taxis, and of course high-quality weed. Mom's health was declining, which made me her primary caregiver, and I'm proud that *she never spent a minute in a nursing home* or a cent on a caregiver, something many *financially secure* families cannot say. These days, people get paid for being a relative's caregiver, as they should.

The highlight film is extensive, with mostly losses in litigation and wins everywhere else, except of course for Banned4Life, who died in March, 2007, and Mom, whose last breath was taken on Thursday, July 26, 2007 at 4:58 a.m.:

- PAP began having spectacular days in 2003, which continued through 2007, and the loss of a seven-percent rebate through Pinnacle, who had also become the bookie of choice for sharp players everywhere, where *slow pay* meant fifteen minutes, not bankruptcy.

- In 2002, the *Ray Gordon Super Bowl Exacta* was offered by Heritage Sports, an elite, under-the-radar bookie who gave me $200.00 in free bets, which I almost turned into $10,000.00 by boxing the Eagles and Patriots, only to have the Rams come back to win after trailing at the half, not realizing I could have picked up four figures with a hedge, and even hit both wagers, but in-game betting was not as mature as it is now.

- Also in 2002, I made *$8,500.00* from a single day of recording a PG-13 audio hypnosis file (*Hellen II*) with a female college student who was able to make her car payments without having to divert time from her studies to a job at *Wal-Mart*. She made as much as me, as the royalties were split 50-50, having agreed to do the work once I guaranteed her a minimum royalty of $500.00, another example of the time portfolio paying dividends. This was a one-time windfall due to difficulty finding specialized talent, and the advent of video, as well as much more talented scriptwiters than me.

- In late 2002, I was diagnosed with Stage III COPD and given five to seven years to live.

- My weekly routine minimized the impact of litigation. As a paralegal, I spent money only on filing fees and supplies, and added a stop at the courthouse on the way to picking up my tapes a few blocks away, near Society Hill, usually on Thursday or Friday. This allowed me to have my day in court with even the largest companies or universities in the world; I avoided smaller targets due to the unfairness of litigation for those without resources, yet was mocked by only picking fair fights rather than extorting settlements.

- In 2004, my final temp assignment landed me in Center City for a video transcription gig which helped me expand into that market, resulting in a steady income after Mom died. I would often transcribe corporate tradeshow interviews, or indie films, which made me feel intellectually superior. This was a Smarty Jones documentary, a horse who attracted 8,000 people to Philadelphia Park (now *Parx Racing*) for a pre-Belmont workout, all by word of mouth. In another example of compounding interests, the video showed modern training technology, including an indoor treadmill on which a horse could run forty-five miles an hour, which I immediately realized meant that first-time starters needed to be judged on the increase in sale price over the sire's stud fee (a *pinhooker*), as their form was hidden.

- The few extra winners the above first-timer angle yielded several mega-exotic wins (like pick-three, pick-four, or superfecta). In 2006, I won so much money that I couldn't even count it, spending it left and right, all thanks to the rebates at Pinnacle. In late 2004, unfortunately, Better Talk Now (26-1) hockey-checked Powerscourt in the Breeders' Cup Turf, with the resulting non-disqualification costing me about $150,000.00 in wins, and literally wiping me out of $100.00 or so. I recovered quickly, however, on the rebate gravy train.

- In 2007, Pinnacle and then Neteller withdrew from the United States market, ending PowerBase and my rebates, mere days after Mom and I each won $600.00+ on an eight-team parlay, thanks to a buzzer-beating three-pointer in overtime by a 2½-point favorite (she just copied my bets into her account). Not long after that, Banned and Mom died, four months apart, leaving me alone in the horseplaying world, and more on my own in the real one. Fortunately, my video transcription business took off, effectively saving me for a few years.

- My employment lawsuits led nowhere. UPenn even got a court-ordered *psychiatric examination* to determine my "employability as a secretary, even as one of their top doctors was imprisoned for drugging and raping a female job applicant." I had a few interviews for office jobs at UPenn that led nowhere, but they continued to be a valued client for transcription and Ph.D. thesis work, particularly their law school (!). Once, their President's office paid my rush rate of $50.00 an hour for a same-day transcript. My internet haters were gleeful to see me discredited, yet ignored that two subsequent requests for exams were denied. I was fined $1,000.00 for defying the order, which triggered a default on my credit-cards, paradoxically increasing my cash flow as I stopped paying.

- The PUA community went mainstream, first through a *New York Times* article by Neil Strauss in 2004, then *The Game*, whose publicity tour was truncated by Hurricane Katrina, and finally *VH-1's The Pickup Artist*, which premiered shortly after Mom died in 2007. As I was not credited for the pivot, nor named like several other gurus, no windfalls resulted, but I did get a nice spike in sales and interest from others.

- Four months before Mom died, two letters were sent to my dying mother, intercepted by me but shown to her, threatening "legal consequences" for her about which they were *seriously concerned*, a phrase used by many who dox those whose speech they do not like, due to her providing me with a place to live and the ability to speak freely on the internet, even though by then I was paying most of the bills and providing end-of-life care. The second letter referenced my landlord and neighbors, showing a clear intent to harass me in my home, all the while Mom was still managing the front desk and working the overnight shift. This ***cyberterrorism*** was completely ignored by law enforcement.

- In 2008, my eyesight began deteriorating due to cataracts which I could not afford to fix. By 2014, I would be legally blind, with vision of ***"WHAT eye chart?"*** In 2019, I had surgery to restore my vision to 20/25, and do not need reading glasses, despite a warning that I would.

- In early 2009, my pulse-ox rose to 95, eliminating the death sentence; I have now had stage III COPD for twenty-two years. It was only here that I quit smoking, due to cost, having continued because, like Patrick Swayze, I saw no point in quitting as it was too late. Apparently, this is not unheard of, but very uncommon.

- Also in early 2009, I won a case when a credit-card company that was suing me dropped the lawsuit after I argued "contributory negligence," i.e., that it was their fault for lending money to me, an argument similar to that used in foreclosure hearings during the financial crisis. I then settled a copyright case with Yahoo! and Microsoft over their search-engine caches, which were eliminated soon after, a result rarely cited by my internet haters.

The internet was hopeless at this point, except for trading and betting, which became my primary uses for it, and interacting with the occasional PUA reader, or gambler.

The Magic Twenty

After Mom died, I stumbled along, until I lost my transcription gig in 2009, leaving me without a steady income. Not panicked, but not knowing what the future would bring, I diverted my last $20.00 from a haircut to handicapping Philadelphia Park on Barack Obama's Inauguration Day. After shaving my head (a tradition which began here, and which saves $80.00 a year), I sat down to make PAP ratings, as I had been doing to document the method for an upcoming book, while putting the finishing touches on ***Understanding And Seducing The Social-Climbing Slut***, the working title for ***Bettor Off Single***.

At 11:45 a.m., I shut off the television due to the distraction, focusing completely on the card, which I almost swept, taking all horizontals except the pick-three in races 2-4, and winding up with $2,583.60 at the end of the card, finally shattering my record for best day from when I found the ticket at Monmouth in 1983, making my best day for over a quarter-century the product of pure luck. I would break this record twice within the next two weeks, as the ***Magic $20.00*** bill had mushroomed into $13,000.00+, which I used as an advance to write ***Bettor Off Single***. That this windfall came during the financial crisis, and my "betters" demanded a ***bailout*** to prevent me from winning, effectively neutralizing my cash just when it was most valuable, was both telling and frustrating, turning me overnight into a hardcore socialist at the very moment I was actually ***winning*** under capitalism, only to have the new losers rig the game with bailouts.

Five:
The Dark Ages And New Light

By the end of 2009, my holding pattern deteriorated, and my need to remain where I was had vanished, since Mom was gone. What followed was a liter and figurative dark age, with my eyesight leaving me (pending cataract surgery), only for me to find a drug that restored it for a few years in 2015, but also a black hole of sorts, into which I retreated. The highlight film was mostly negative, though the time portfolio was holding up just fine. Any bright spots were horribly overshadowed, as I approached the half-century mark:

- For the remainder of 2009, I lost back a good deal of my winnings, in search of jackpots, but still had a nice profit by the end of the year.

- Also in 2009, *incel* George Sodini killed three women at an L.A. Fitness center, igniting the feminist backlash to PUA that continues to this day against the likes of Andrew Tate and others, and will no doubt only change form in the future, without ever ending.

- From 2010-2012, I released a half-dozen or so PUA books, and a dozen or more chess books, most of which sold some copies, and continue to have an audience to this day. In 2015, I retired from the genre, due to no longer wishing to intrude in the personal lives of my readers, and to increase my focus in chess, now that I had enough of my eyesight back and it seemed I'd be around a while.

- In 2011, a single PUA student found me online, praised my work, and said he had poor results with the other gurus. Within four years he no longer needed advice, and paid me relatively well. It was nice to still cash in on work I had done many years earlier, with ongoing potential to cash in, for yet another dividend check from my "wasted youth."

- In 2012, I dismissed Bitcoin at $1.00 because I figured mine would be hacked or deleted, plus I didn't think crypto would go anywhere. The number of bitcoin millionaires created during the boom is testimony to people who wound up wealthy by believing in a cause rather than chasing money for its own sake.

- In 2015, I was diagnosed with cirrhosis of the liver and type II diabetes, both ultimately terminal illnesses, and wound up on Social Security Disability (SSDI), two months before my work experience would have become stale, leaving me on the draconian SSI. In 2021, I was diagnosed with end-stage liver disease and given only a year to live. I am currently functional but increasingly fragile and more likely to die at any time. A transplant can extend my life expectancy by allowing me to die twice!

- In 2018, I left the only home I had known since 1987, save for brief discount sublets in the area (or Brooklyn in 1988), and the four months in Albany, Georgia in 2000. I wound up homeless for a bit, then finally stabilized in Chinatown, Philadelphia, and will likely have moved on before you have read this. My time here has been relatively uneventful, providing an excellent place for *alpha isolation*, where money is now my top priority, with my only goals as a chessplayer to cement my legacy by finishing my work on the *tunnel* opening method, and making my retirement as financially lucrative as possible, while enjoying the rewards of the time portfolio that have only increased, and which leaves me with never a dull moment.

- In 2019, sports betting was legalized in Pennsylvania, along with medical marijuana. Congress made an honest man of me, as I could now openly enjoy my favorite pastimes, and do. PowerBase has resurged, with great jackpot potential, including a 40-1 win on Florida Atlantic to make the Final Four in 2022, a windfall made possible only by a software written thirty years ago while on a "dead end job."

- Also in 2019, I defeated GM Anton Korobov, the #42-ranked player in the world, rated 2688 FIDE, at one-minute chess, in fifteen moves, with Black, in a ***Queen's Gambit Accepted*** (QGA). The advent of online play, the Netflix series, and the COVID pandemic created a perfect storm which turned chess literally overnight into a billion-dollar sport. I then contemplated quitting chess, figuring I'd never top this, and while I haven't quit, I haven't come close to this, other than the victory over Tariq Yue.

- Changes in the statute of limitations for child sex-abuse cases opened a window for lawsuits that let me file a ***$2.6 million*** claim over an incident in 1984. Suffice it to say the outcome was not that lucrative, but having a lawyer was worth it as she had my back in numerous places. Litigation is generally a waste of time and should be used only as a last resort.

- In March, 2020, I wound up locked down in the COVID pandemic, and survived. I have had seven vaccinations, with the only side effect that my left arm felt like I had pitched nine innings of MLB.

Over the past decade, commissions on stocks and options have been reduced to nothing or nearly nothing, while the proliferation of 0dte options makes all other gambling games irrelevant. Unprecedented opportunity now exists, which is why my time alternates between daytrading SPX options and chess, plus using PowerBase for sports betting, which takes very little time and requires no babysitting; I usually check the results at the end of the night, unless it's a ***Big Game*** like the Super Bowl. My health is certainly a concern, and I won't be alive for most of my audience for this work, as many more will find me only after I'm gone, a normal occurrence online, where delayed fame is also extremely common due to the sheer volume of content and the ease with which it can be produced.

Six:
Bring Something To Do

Staying the course and prioritizing my interests outside of work, while using my office career to gain deep knowledge of white-collar America and its professional niches, is the only reason I can sit here at fifty-seven, half-dead, and still have a chance not just to survive, but to thrive financially, while thriving every day I awaken able to play chess online, daytrade, bet sports or DFS, bingewatch a show like *Frasier*, which I missed while maximizing my twenties, and retaining a ***time portfolio*** which cannot be seized in bankruptcy. Indeed, the ***jackpot potential*** offered by this portfolio, as evidenced by the Florida Atlantic win, and many other futures bets, is immune even to the inevitable medical bankruptcies which swallow whole those who do not die early or quickly enough. The ***Estate Recovery Act*** then cleans out what's left of the estate, rendering all that youthful sacrifice not just moot, but self-destructive.

SPX options are so lucrative and life-changing that the ability to pick them dwarfs everything else in determining someone's lot in life. On a daily basis, wagers as small as $5.00 can become ***$4,000.00+*** in a matter of hours, while ten-baggers in half a day or even an hour are routine. This was not available until recently, indicating the importance of timing in your retirement planning, as well as other life decisions, like marriage, which led to the ***#mtgow*** movement of men who once earned far more than me, yet who wind up broke in middle age, not even making it to retirement, while I'm just finding my stride.

A Day In The Life

For however much time I have left, I spend my days playing chess online (managed ***225 games*** in a single day recently!), and in the occasional tournament, though after I beat Tariq Yue I felt I had proven the tunnel effective in tournament play. I make YouTube videos when I have something to say, and livestream my chess once in a while to demonstrate my method and current progress. As of this writing, my peak LiChess one-minute rating is 2337, in a chess world infinitely more robust than in Fischer's day, where a single tournament win is now more difficult than contending for the title way back when. I am now three generations removed from the pre-engine era, when few players took the game seriously, to an environment more like golf and tennis, so loaded with talent that everyone in the top few percentiles stands out. Anyone who wants my chess work can download it free of charge via links on my YouTube channel or social-media profiles.

Capitalism makes compulsive gamblers out of all of us, while the lack of basic income and a social safety net ensures that most of us will wind up broke in old age, with only our pensions or social security benefits as a cushion, but an excellent one at that. The system accomplishes its primary goal of preventing elderly poverty, and I certainly would be lost without my benefits, achieved through almost thirty years of fulltime employment, with many of my years not credited due to the exemption for family businesses. Through my teens, I was one of the highest-earning children not in sports or entertainment, all by dint of my own initiative. My parents were true hustlers, always chasing the next windfall or opportunity, and having an incredible time along the way. Working on Merzie's books and playing chess against elite prodigies in my old age offer experiences and value that money can't buy, and they become much more rewarding when prioritized throughout one's life.

When writing this text, in the space of the few days I could spare to leave a final mark on the world, I realized that ***intellectual dishonesty*** is the true poison, rendering fake, irrelevant, and downright misleading what we used to rely on as shortcuts to navigate through life. The underpinnings of this trust have been obliterated by unapologetic sociopathy, from people who act incredulous when Charlie Brown elects not to kick the football. Many of my haters will have little if any legacy at all, because they spent their time anonymously attacking people, while leaving nothing of value to future audiences. While I cannot speculate where I'll wind up in history, I know my work has already impacted the world in a way few will ever experience, in large part due to timing and circumstance rather than any conscious effort to become famous. I would much rather have quietly gotten rich and married a beauty queen.

I cannot tell you how to live your life, but I can say that a nest egg goes only so far, and that true wealth in retirement comes as much from your achievements and how you occupy your time rather than the size of your nest egg, which is not likely to last as long as you think it will, and once that happens, you're going to have a lot of time, which means you should not only bring something to do, but take time throughout your life to make sure you do it well. This approach to life, rather than being preoccupied with money the system rarely allows the elderly to keep, has ensured I am never bored, and still relevant in niches where I do more than merely pass time. I couldn't ask for a better retirement, however long it may last. I take each day God gives me, and make the absolute most of it, which shows up most in my chess rating, the result of a lifetime of the productive investment of one's time.

Once I'm gone, my ideas will live on, while the self-interest that defines temporal debate will vanish, along with my ability to continue my work. It is my hope that the next generation picks up where I left off. Another upside to options trading or being able to multiply money, as well as being on a fixed income, is that I don't ***need*** money, which frees me to release everything into the wild (except this text!). At that point everything is out of my hands, and the rest is up to you, the reader. It's not my place to tell history what to do with my legacy, only to leave it for anyone who wishes to continue by putting their own stamp on my ideas. For all I have endured, which is but a fraction of the worst injustice inflicted on others, the positives have more than outweighed the negative, while allowing me the opportunity for creative fulfillment, while living the dream of those who buy lottery tickets, but with better winning chances.

Moral Hazard: You Are What You F**k

You can't win a game when your opponent is also the referee. Women, and their "simps," operate as if they were the NFL replay booth of sex: ***"after further review…"*** If the ***way*** a man gets laid does not meet with the approval of the replay committee (everyone within earshot of her complaints or praise), the sex is retroactively nullified, at times to the point of being redefined as harassment or rape. While ***false allegations*** make for sensational headlines, and most definitely destroy the lives of innocent men, women have infinite ways of accomplishing this; the root of that problem is men's desire for sex, which creates the much larger problem of ***rewarding bad behavior***, which makes the behavior seem good, solely because women reward it with sex!! This makes high-earning men declare themselves winners, which in turn creates a world where self-worth equates to net worth, where character takes a backseat to greed, all because ***<u>women trade sex for money</u>***, either directly or indirectly.

Women justify their ***hypergamy*** out of pure self-interest: no one is going to pay her bills, while she is in demand among men. This results in men being judged financially, as I was on Walnut Street by my former neighbor, whose opinion of the lawyer she married and of me was strictly financial, and she was the only one who verbalized what many other women were too polite to express, forcing ***them*** to invent character defects to justify their rejection, intellectual dishonesty enforced by insults, ostracization, and even doxing, harassment, and death threats to men who step out of line by speaking the simple truth, as the PUA community learned then, and as Andrew Tate and his followers are learning now, though the modern weapon is ***deplatforming***, which kickstarted the community in the 1990s when AOL banned people like me for "misogyny" while allowing open season on the male point of view.

Rather than complain about women wanting men with money, I invite them to reconsider how they measure wealth. That I am thriving in retirement should have been expected, just as it was for Murph, whose military benefits and other retirement perks kicked in, stabilizing his finances, which allowed his chess to thrive, both as a nationally renowned coach, and as a player who is now top five in the country in blitz, as his age peers retire. Even at fifty-seven, my rating is moving me up the age lists, though I don't acknowledge ***senior chess***, instead considering myself a senior who plays chess, but the reality is that I no longer have to be a champion to leave a mark, the bar lowering every year I stay alive. By the ***We Are Marshall*** metric, I "won" my game against Tariq Yue just by showing up still able to make the trip and play a top prodigy.

If women decided tomorrow that money didn't matter, the wealthy men who believe themselves superior would be laughed at as unattractive, overweight, and extremely boring in most cases, yet attach a six-figure income to this man and he's suddenly a ***good catch***, while men like me are downplayed for not being ***financially secure***, just because I don't meet a narrow, indirect definition of wealth. From there, verbal abuse almost seems justified, almost as social pressure to conform to a nonexistent ideal. Any attempt to defend my lifestyle or point out flaws in how they judge others is met with further appeals to stereotype in order to discredit my argument, such as calling me a loser who lives with Mom even if I had sex on my rooftop with a woman who laughed at them earlier that evening in a bar.

As for ***#defundwomen***, men who complain either about the price of sex, or their inability to get laid, are funding their own demise by giving money to women with whom they are not having sex. The woman who can start a patronage page can get money directly from her adoring audience for nothing but a few ***PG-13 pictures***, as if they still had value, which they apparently will until the market crashes, at which point they'll up the ante, with hotter women doing more to stand out, much like during the financial crisis, when high-level secretaries in Manhattan resorted to stripping and turning tricks.

Garbage Conversations

The cancer of intellectual dishonesty permeates all human interaction, rendering most of it worthless, or what I call ***garbage conversations***, where either one of two people is conning the other, or a pair of ignorant people find a like mind. Somewhere, some Nigerian scammer is pretending to be a Prince, while their stateside target is excitedly awaiting their $20 million wire transfer. In 1995, when I was winning like clockwork with PowerBase, a bartender at my local tavern told me about his "insider connections" (a scamdicapper) who was going to help him win betting sports; I tried to assist with PowerBase, but he was all-in, hook, line and sinker; a few months later he was in distress and bankrupt.

Without thinking, we allow the intellectually dishonest to *engage* us, meeting my expanded definition of *sealioning*, like the time in 1987 a beginner at chess made me stand outside in the cold rain on my skates, late in the evening, for forty minutes to finish him off from a winning position, which I did out of sheer stubbornness, in part as an ambassador of the game, but also as a test of my professionalism, and I passed. Back then, to the public, especially women, I was *ChessDude*, their window on the chess world, with my expert's rating commanding respect. Fast-forward to today, and she's seen *The Queen's Gambit*, can check my rating online, and will find a chess world populated by thousands of players who train as hard as Fischer, unlike then. I am no longer unique in that regard.

Many of my garbage conversations were in job interviews where employers had to invent pretexts not to hire me, with UPenn taking this to the extreme by declaring me *unemployable*, even while I was employed as a psych transcriptionist (!) For years, I had heard that I was overqualified, yet was never offered the supposedly superior position that should have been mine. Eventually, I realized that intellectual dishonesty is so toxic that I avoid it at all costs, terminating any interaction with people at the first sign of it, because conversations with these people are useless, designed to persuade and gaslight by exploiting our tendency to treat them as sharing useful information, much like my 1986 haters wanted me to believe they were being helpful when advising me not to "waste my life at the track," when in reality they were just trying to cause a *tilt* that would stop my winning streak.

At the track, I went from letting haterz chill my optimism in 1986, to laughing at them in 1991, which in two cases led to threats of violence from people who couldn't stand to see me win. In employment, I began to see the gaslighting for what it was in 1993, and became a whistleblower and activist, causing employers to escalate to blacklisting and declaring me *unemployable* in open court, while an intellectually dishonest world stands down, all the while implying that something were wrong with me, yet claiming I have ***issues*** if I avoid them.

Chess is a game of perpetual gaslighting: players sell unsound openings as sound, and not resigning losing positions they pass off as playable. Those who tell us not to listen to others throw the biggest fits when we tune them out. Chess publishing is also built on intellectual dishonesty, with ridiculously expensive, voluminous courses that don't help players improve touted as required reading, validated by strong players who are all paid to promote the system. Even tournament chess is intellectually dishonest: instead of using e-sport arcades that don't require travel, they hold events in expensive hotels, for free playing space in exchange for filling the hotel with players, and the games are at slow time controls, not because they produce better chess, but to fill the hotel over a long weekend, rather than a single afternoon or evening, that could even be held in a restaurant in between the lunch and dinner rush.

Consider the implications of the censorship I faced from the PUA community, with some commercial interests literally *commandeering* the group through its FAQ, which is supposed to set norms for the group, not direct them to an external website that has an owner, practices censorship, and which is not archived, in this case resulting in several years of history being erased once the site removed its archives. *mASF* had begun as a searchable USENET archive during the eighteen months Google took down the AltaVista archive prior to rebranding it as *Google Groups*, itself a bit misleading, because USENET is not a Google property, and would exist fine without them. To build an entire website based on excluding me shows the lengths to which some will go to suppress dissent or control a narrative, a problem which only worsened in the ensuing quarter-century.

Through my individual pastimes, I avoid almost all intellectual dishonesty, and have trained myself to recognize it immediately, so I don't waste time on misinformation or those who spread it, either out of ignorance or hidden malice. Social trust has been exploited by sociopaths who rely on our good nature, and our belief that others wouldn't be so self-destructive as to burn the bridge with a single betrayal. Absent this trait, I'd have been little more than a ***basic bitch***, a man who thinks he's doing everything right because ***they*** agree with him, yet who loses out to independent thinkers, like the ones who found Bitcoin in 2011 and took the plunge, who figured out that marriage is best avoided (***#mgtow***), and who didn't follow the crowd, though by definition, contrarians will always be in the minority.

* * *

I will conclude with a series of essays on various topics related to the text, and society at large. Intellectual dishonesty has rendered public debate meaningless as anything but a propaganda tool. In the 1990s, the internet was so starved for content that anyone who produced almost anything made it big, or at least a nice extra income, as I did, but it didn't last, as Big Tech became its self-appointed gatekeeper, beginning with censorship on AOL once they gained market dominance. AOL used to have ***guides*** patrolling its chats, booting people for even a single curse word, or for, as on ***Netgirl***, "offending women." We clamor for honest debate about hot-button topics yet refuse to allow the free expression they require, particularly if any negative truths about women are involved.

This text outlines my blueprint for dealing with intellectual dishonesty, and those who either bully others, or stand down as witnesses. That others don't recognize the problem, let alone try to solve it, goes a long way towards revealing how the current state of the world, and the internet, resolved. As one who believes that ***small minds discuss people***, I have deliberately avoided namechecking or calling out anyone specific, because once we die, our petty disputes with others give way to our legacy, in my case chess, PowerBase, PUA, dating advice, MGTOW, and political activism relating to ***#metoo***, affirmative action, and gender discrimination, with two lawsuits mentioned on the front pages of ***The Wall Street Journal*** and ***New York Times***. Perhaps death will amplify my voice in a way Big Tech refused to.

Essay #1:
Lifestyle Integration (Side Hustles)

Hustle culture, exemplified by FIRE, says life is a hustle that should end only after you've achieved *Financial Independence* so you can *Retire Early,* or think you're retired until old age wipes out even your seven-figure nest egg. While I can't say I *chose* to maximize my twenties, as FIRE was my first plan, employment discrimination relegated me to the type of jobs held by people who will either get nowhere in life, or who have a very rich life outside of work, like *Mr. Shaibel.* Ironically, the school at which I coached chess for a semester had a janitor who was a jazz historian with a popular local radio show, and was much more interesting than the "sexy" white-collar men women line up to marry. Indeed, if women were to suddenly say money didn't matter, most of these men wouldn't care about money. Enter *lifestyle integration*, a way of maximizing your time portfolio.

When I was offered the overnight concierge desk shift in late 1987, it was a perfect opportunity to train at chess, yielding a paycheck for doing in my lobby what I had already been doing upstairs. Over the years, I would also use this job, which covered my basic expenses, to write books like *Outfoxing The Foxes*, programs like PowerBase, or to make speed figures. When I was working in Center City, Mom would greet me at the end of her shift with a prepared *Racing Form* that allowed me to wager on my lunch hour while working a job only one block from the Center City Turf Club, which I had taken for that reason, after quitting an indefinite assignment at Temple University Hospital because it was three miles away.

In retrospect, I could have wagered over the phone while at Temple, but I wanted to work in Center City, and for the big law firm that hired me in December, under the *intellectually dishonest* pretext of "temp to perm," when in reality they were cutting staff and just using me to cover for all the **_women_** in support positions. Seeing female high-school students still in uniform as they exited law offices at 5:00 p.m., or seeing firsthand how they were hired and then harassed when working for neighboring firms to my employers, made the *#metoo* problem obvious, many years before anyone was "woke." The front desk was a refuge, one which allowed me to fully explore my creative and entrepreneurial sides, with what are now called *side hustles*.

Each decision to integrate my lifestyle for maximum time efficiency paid off incredibly. Even in retirement, I "crop rotate" by playing chess while waiting for trading or betting results, saving time with bots written thirty years ago in Paradox, which I integrated into my office work by getting paid to train on it, and seeking jobs which required it for three years, until Windows took over. This text is another example of integration, as it is more or less a stream-of-consciousness rant that makes use of my downtime from chess or other activities. The goal of lifestyle integration is to maximize opportunity and time-efficiency, while eliminating boredom.

Anyone can practice lifestyle integration: a construction worker might invest in rehabilitating properties for rental or resale, effectively monetizing his existing skills, while a struggling musician (or chessplayer) might also publish or teach, though I never did that because I was trying to become a champion. Andrew Beyer had excellent lifestyle integration between his paycheck, wagering, and later his contract with the *Racing Form* to be their speed-figure provider. Not fixating on one's nest egg, or retirement, opens up many possibilities, and gives financial motivation that comes with not having money to burn, or thinking you do even if few keep their money for very long in old age.

Essay #2:
Trading Places

Want to turn **_$5.00 into $4,000.00 in three hours?_** Not only is this possible, but it's a daily occurrence on Wall Street. I watched it happen right before my eyes, with an option I sold for $0.15 to save money (I did make about $200.00 on another wager), usually wise late in the day, as these options rarely recover, but when they do the results are spectacular. This incredible level of opportunity has changed the American landscape to where it rewards compulsive gambling even more now than ever, to the point where every human on the planet should see if they can make a living trading SPX options, or their poor relative, the SPY (basically 10 percent of SPX).

If God indeed had a plan for me, my lifetime of betting horses and sports was preparation for the big leagues: daytrading of **_zero days to expiration_** (0dte) SPX options, which are tied to the **_Standard & Poor 500_** Index, a key economic benchmark. The SPY is an ETF (exchange-traded fund), billed in the 1990s as **_"the entire S&P 500, in a single stock."_** In reality, about a quarter of the ETF is invested in the largest big-caps, and the index itself is not a stock at all, which makes SPX options **_bets_** little more than large-scale gambling; **_VERY_** large-scale gambling, of the kind that allows for **_rollups_** which put anything I've ever done to shame. A smart woman would check her man's ability to predict the SPX rather than looking at his bank account, but most still use traditional, outdated metrics.

While I sometimes share my opinions on the SPX – the only thing I trade – Wall Street is the one domain where I do not freely share my information, but also the reason everything else I do is free and/or demonetized (i.e., commercial-free). I did set up Snodgrass Publishing Group to retain the rights to my work, over which I have complete control, and have a kindle store for people who want to put my books on their readers, but most are available free by PDF, in part because options trading is where I seek wealth, and because my disability check means I'm already getting paid a **_basic income_**, so I am hardly uncompensated. This has freed me to maximize my audience and refrain from trying to **_sell_** my ideas, instead letting nature take its course without the barrier to entry of high cost.

Intellectual dishonesty is rampant in financial markets, from investors and analysts who deliberately mislead the masses to cash in on the other side of the trades, to **_influenzers_** who make money with courses and videos that teach people what they think they already know. My immunity to gaslighters and other timewasters allows me instead to code my bot, and let it ruthlessly build an edge similar to the one I still enjoy with PowerBase, which puts me in a position to win **_life-changing or generational wealth_**, literally from scratch (just like 1983 and 2009), but on a much larger scale, with the benefit of tax advantages (rebates!), and the lack of stigma, with many even seeking advice on how to trade, as one stripper did when she knocked down her paywall to pick my brain at her club, which might have led somewhere had she not taken a regular job.

Thanks to Dad's training, **_alarm bells_** go off when I see jackpots, and SPX is a daily, ongoing jackpot that makes even bitcoin or PowerBall/Megamillions pale by comparison. The average person buys lottery tickets hoping to win, but also for the mental exercise of planning how to spend money they **_might_** win, and the "lesser" prizes, which are very hittable, are certainly nothing to sneeze at. If I were a lottery degenerate, however, I would sell tickets, hoping to score the $100,000.00 bonus or whatever it is now for selling a jackpot ticket, while collecting six percent or whatever they pay out of each ticket sold.

In another example of lifestyle integration, some professional horseplayers purchased an OTB that allowed them to keep the track's share of the takeout as a betting rebate – the edge that chased me away from the track, even before Maple Leaf Mel. Back in the days when sports betting was illegal, and commissions too expensive, the track played a vital role in both my time and betting portfolio, but has since been rendered obsolete. Rebates were not as much of an issue until the past decade, when the effects of long-term cannibalism of the recreational players has made it next to impossible to win, except on big days, and even then way too much handicapping work is required.

For as much as I once loved the track, I love profitability and not wasting time even more, so the track was left behind for SPX. Sports betting and DFS have replaced them in my portfolio, but in each case I use algorithms and bots to eliminate the need for handicapping, allowing me to handicap and place my bets in minutes a day, yielding hours of enjoyment, profits, and a significant amount of *free money* whenever a bookie is offering a bonus, particularly new ones for new customers. With bots that can churn a bankroll and break even or better, rollover requirements are not an issue.

Intellectually Dishonest Financial Advice

Public ignorance of investing runs so deep that misinformation and disinformation are the norm:

- ♦ ***You can't time the market.*** Wall Street's answer to ***you can't beat the races*** discourages people from doing the one thing which might make the wealthy, and which is wrong. Maybe ***you*** can't time the market, but successful traders have to or they would go bankrupt. Intraday movement that have very little to do with investing, but can still be analyzed like any wager. A 0dte SPX option can go from \$1.00 to \$12.00 in an hour, then back to zero an hour later; it is the wildest, most profitable betting option ever invented, with little or no rake, vigorish, commissions, or house edge. A sharp gambler adapts, even if it means abandoning a game one loves, as I should have done with harness racing in 1980, but did not until 1986.

- ♦ ***You can't beat the races***. This drum was beaten into my brain from childhood, by anyone who saw me with binoculars around my neck and a ***Racing Form***, in an era where one could not hide their wagering from the world, as they can now. In 1991, I could not avoid the Turf Club and still keep my job. Winning money in a small room crowded with losing bettors is a recipe for conflict. Thankfully, within a few short years I was able to wager online, bypassing PhoneBet altogether, which of course led to them unbanning me (Sol seemed to have something to do with that). My last big ***rollup*** at the track was \$4.50 into \$1,000.00+ in an hour on Breeders' Cup day, 2019, after which the pandemic, then Maple Leaf Mel, ended my interest in the sport.

- ♦ ***Take profits!*** With the 0.05 SPX option that went to 41.00, I sold at around 2.20, following the "sound" advice to lock in profits, thus costing myself almost four dimes. While I agree that avoiding ruin is paramount, there is no inherent advantage in profit-taking, or bailing on a losing trade, as evidenced by this one's rebound from 0.05 (I had bought at around 0.35). Late in the day, SPX goes truly ***bats**t***, where nickels, dimes and quarters can turn into dead presidents you've long forgotten on denominations which exist only in a bank vault. Why, then doesn't anyone get rich doing this? They do…*once*, after which they are already rich.

- ♦ ***Options Are Too Risky***. Actually, options cut risk a lot by using leverage, and avoids disaster when a stock plummets, as many do after earnings or news, some gaining or losing half their value rapidly. Since most investors sell their losers after a 10-15 percent drop, they are not even betting their own bankroll, but rather functioning as their own margin lender, hoping to gain the power of a $1,000 trade in which they will bail if it drops to $900.00, converting a ten percent loss into a 100 percent loss, when an option would have lost but a fraction of that.

- ◆ ***PDT and other rules are for your own good!*** The pattern-daytrading (PDT) rules are designed to prevent poor people from ***Trading Places*** with the wealthy. The rules apply to anyone with less than $25,000.00, while those above that threshold can make unlimited daytrades. The rule is intellectually dishonest because it is presented "for your own good," much like the ***accredited investors,*** who must have a high net worth to make risky investments, even though anyone can walk into a casino, sportsbook or racetrack without restriction. The best workaround is to use a cash account which allows you unlimited trades up to the balance in the account each day, with options settling overnight, and SPX not even counting as a daytrade if held until cash settlement.

- ◆ ***Don't risk too much of your bankroll.*** This is fine if you are independently wealthy, but ***living expenses count as losses***, putting most of us four figures into the hole on the first of each month, as VegasDude noted in one of his many mentoring e-mails. His existence thumbed its nose at intellectual dishonesty, seeing through it thanks to his birds-eye view of the sports betting subculture, including a national clientele of bookmakers, sharps, and everyone else, including me, thanks to PowerBase opening that door, and of course Sol opening the door to the software that has been my bread-and-butter for over three decades, saving me countless handicapping time, including twenty hours a week of making power ratings the second I finished coding. This primitive AI foreshadowed an era where those who master it can literally print money.

- ◆ ***Don't play options!*** See Keith Gill below for what is possible with options, and consider why someone would leave 99 percent of their profits on the table if they were so sure of their opinion. With living expenses counting as losses, options reduce your infrastructure costs, as does betting as many markets as possible, including sports betting an DFS, assuming you can code a profitable bot (my "secret sauce").

Like those old game shows where only the final round mattered, SPX options now control who controls the money, whether traded directly or as a hedge against the market as a whole. Capitalism makes gamblers out of all of us, even by omission, as those who passed on Bitcoin can attest. Those who become wealthy through trading wind up your employer, landlord, or rival bidder for goods and services, all tangible rewards for the singular skill of handicapping the SPX or the stock market in general, as well as horse racing, sports betting, DFS, and countless other gambling games where billions or even trillions of dollars are moved around each year, all winding up in the hands of the skilled, or the house, relegating to poverty those whose only crime is to not be a ***quant***, or math prodigy with a father who schooled them in kindergarten.

#Fintwit, #WallStreetBets, and Meme Stocks

Netflix's ***Dumb Money*** tells the story of Keith "Roaring Kitty" "DeepF**kingValue" Gill, a Massachusetts financial analyst whose tapout bet on GameStop calls (not shares!) turned his $53,000.00 life savings into almost ***$50 million*** in about a year, with most of the gains in a few weeks. The man who threatened me on AOL was known for taking a few hundred dollars into an options pit and making hundreds of millions. As I learned from ***The Handicapper,*** money follows knowledge, with most of the profits coming at the very end, testing our resolve and ability to deal with intellectually dishonest verbal abuse every step of the way. The meme stocks eventually got slaughtered, in part because the "buy" button was shut down at some brokers, but any bubble will burst; they put the fear of God in Wall Street.

Let me make clear that, aside from a few minor windfalls, I have never gotten rich trading SPX options…*yet*. PowerBase (particularly futures like Florida Atlantic to make the 2023 Final Four at 40-1) is still my best ***option***, and the SPY offers more than enough action with limited (relative) risk, but the ***potential*** for literally anyone to break the bank, as Gill did, is substantial and perpetual. As a ***jackpot hunter***, I tend to reinvest any winnings (after spending some on bills) in search of a life-changing score, of which I need exactly ***one,*** and I continue to work on my bot to figure out this shark tank, with the world's best quants, poker players, gamblers, and everyone else does combat every morning at 9:30, in a tax-advantaged game, socially acceptable game with a reduced takeout.

You don't have to be a hardcore jackpot hunter to make money with options trading, but it's more fun to live the meme stock dream, and SPX offers this opportunity perpetually. Those who wish to dial down risk can toss on some training wheels and try the SPY, which I do in times of uncertainty or a lower bankroll, but this and every name now takes a backseat to ***chess***, which gives me things money cannot purchase (though a jackpot would make logistics easier), such as the win over Tariq Yue, the ability to remain relevant beyond "checkers in a nursing home," and of course a ***legacy*** which is already being built by players like Leon, the 1700 who used the ***tunnel*** to defeat an IM in tournament play. Fortunately, chess and trading and betting are not mutually exclusive, instead ensuring that I am literally never board, and thanks to the bots I don't have to waste time to handicap or trade at the highest levels, instead delegating that to the algos.

I cannot and would not tell you what to do with your money or how to invest. Just like in chess, I tell others that this is the move *I* would play, and explain why, but whichever moves ***you*** want to make are up to you; indeed, I refuse to coach children at chess because they can learn from playing against me in tournaments (Yue saw the value of a bishop pair against double pawns, for example), and because as I also say, they need to learn to play like them rather than play like me. What everyone has in common, however, is the need to recognize intellectual dishonesty and not react to manipulation from someone who may be betting against you. As I say in chess, ***never listen to your opponent.***

Essay #3:
Chess

In 1971, Mom bought me a chess set to keep me occupied while she built Manhattan's largest transcription service, in part because I was a math prodigy, or ***numbers whiz***, as she called it, but also due to the Fischer Boom, which spawned a national chess craze that died out by the end of the decade, but which also gave rise to a longer-term uptick in tournament play, the ***Searching For Bobby Fischer*** generation, and then online play, followed by the rise of streaming, the pandemic, and of course ***The Queen's Gambit***, resulting in a chess world which bears little resemblance to the one in which I grew up. Chess is a game of gaslighting and intellectual dishonesty, where unsound openings are played as if sound, and losing positions are played on as if there were drawing or winning chances, but the holy grail of intellectual dishonesty smacked me in the face when I finally got serious in 1986:

If you are not a master by age twenty-one, you'll never be world champion.

In 1984, the Samford Fellowship was created to incentivize Americans to train for the world title, which drew me in, mostly as a focal point, since my last year of eligibility was 1991 (the Fellowship is for twenty-five and under), at which point I'd check my progress and decide whether or not to make chess a career. For many reasons, including not winning the fellowship (I was never rating-eligible), I quit at age twenty-four, shifted my focus to speed figures, and later PowerBase, and never looked back, save for the occasional session with Murph, who'd stop by on NFL Sunday afternoons for air conditioning, a meal, and to keep my game "tuned," which he did.

In 2015, I returned to a chess world that barely resembled the one I had left, with severe implications for my world-title aspirations, which even to this day cannot be completely ruled out, given the quantum leaps that are possible with a game now nearly completely ***<u>solved</u>*** by engines, with the truth slowly spilling over into human play, through methods like my tunnel, or more traditional repertoires, where engines act like a spellchecker, and which is now very similar to…***PacMan***, a videogame I had solved years earlier, even playing against Bill Bastable's perfect game in July, 1983 at the all-night arcade at Sixty-First and First, which I attested on a video because apparently there's a big internet controversy surrounding who got a perfect score and when; the documentary ***The Perfect Fraudman*** (2012).

While the chess world was dismissing me as I "aged out," it turns out that videogames set the table for the tunnel, and my lifetime peak rating at an age where I'm supposedly well past my prime.

<u>The Hunger Games</u>

My "secret" for solving chess (or attempting to solve it) is rooted in the arcades, which have one key difference from chess:

- In chess, if you make a mistake, you resign (or get checkmated), set up the board, and try again, knowing you will improve over time.

♦ In the arcade, if you make a mistake, you pull a quarter out of your pocket and feed *$0.25 per mistake* into the machine, usually from a teenager's budget (I was making $200.00+ a week working for Mom so this wasn't as much of an issue).

The financial pressure of mistakes in arcade gaming instilled a level of perfectionism unrivaled in chess, reflected in the latter's tolerance for imperfect play that would bankrupt the typical arcade gamer in hours. I know this to be true because this pressure was nonexistent on my *Atari* home system, which I never mastered because not doing so didn't empty my pockets. This was completely lost on the chess world, who in 1987 saw only a washed-up, twenty-year-old, rather than an experienced videogamer with a highly relevant skillset, thanks to *tunnel*-vision that did not acknowledge my strengths, which have only been amplified in the engine era, and which resulted in a total lack of respect, no funding, and downright *mocking* from others which shows that chess is as close to a *caste system* as we have in America. As it turned out, not a single Fellowship winner from the 1980s became world champion, and now so many players are funded that it would be a surprise for that to continue.

To be fair, I didn't quit chess in 1991 because of social pressure, but the Fellowship would certainly have kept me on that path. I quit instead because the Beyer method had a limited shelf life, with the *Daily Racing Form* picking up his speed figures, and while they were in *The Racing Times*, even that minor expense was too much for many for a method which had become common currency. In the months before I got *Banned4Life* from the Turf Club, the track was like a supermarket shopping spree, with limited time to cash in, and cash in we did. Mom and I paid taxes on around $40,000.00 in winnings in 1990-1991 alone, and after 1992, almost nothing, but fortunately PowerBase picked up the slack until PAP kicked in around 1998. The other problem was that my *tunnel* method for chess required perfect play from engines, which I expected around 2003 at age thirty-six, rather than 2019, at fifty-two, another example of how timing is beyond our control.

Beating My Friends (1971-1984)

Unlike most chess prodigies, whose careers are planned by parents who live vicariously through them, Mom and Dad couldn't have cared any less about my progress, or whether or not I won, as they wanted me to pursue my own interests, and figured I would likely succeed at whatever I did. As long as I kept my grades up I could pretty much do what I wanted. The highlight film is rather bare, yet also laid the groundwork for my highly independent and unique approach to the game:

♦ After a few months, Mom and Dad refused to play me, because I beat them every time.

♦ In fourth grade, I beat WaiterDude (from *Bettor Off Single*) three times in a row, to become the P.S. 158 lunchroom champion, a title we would trade back and forth all year. My opponent had studied theory, which influenced my play, mostly based on tactics. Without reading any books, I had taught myself knight forks, skewers, pins, and discovered check. To this day, I can envision a knight's path between any two squares on the board.

♦ In seventh grade, my science teacher showed me the Philidor Defense as an example of a top opening, but the lesson was lost on me, to the point where the concept of an opening repertoire didn't even register, as I was too preoccupied with pinball, videogames, and the track. Chess was what I played when someone pushed me in front of board (because math prodigy), in bad weather when I couldn't go outside, or in the evenings when we didn't have enough for poker or

Monopoly, the latter the worst board game ever created, and not even a game at all, but an equation that highlights the evils of capitalism.

♦ In August, 1981, I played chess for a few hours in Washington Square Park, where I met Ralph the Hustler, a large, imposing man with a chess game to match. When asked to play a ten-game set at $2.00 a game, I declined, not having to prove that I'd lose all ten. Ralph was 2300 strength or so, his main talents keeping order in the chess tables set up by hustlers on Manhattan streets, and cherry-picking his opponents.

♦ In October, 1981, I encountered Jackie Beers, childhood friend of Bobby Fischer, on the track bus back from Roosevelt, giving us more than an hour to kill. Beers regaled me with tales of Fischer's childhood, and how he'd sit in the *Automat* at Grand Central in the overnights, playing all comers for fifty cents a game, and beating them without even looking up from his *New York Times*. I told Beers I was a *chess master*, the title given to me by Wagner when I won the school championship, but I was not the 2200+ prodigy he thought. Beers suggested we play sometime, and eventually we did, in the first round of the 1987 National Chess Congress, to a draw, but he was tired after a long trip down.

♦ The 1978 and 1981 matches between Karpov and Korchnoi ended the Fischer Boom, as chess reverted to a game dominated by interchangeable Russians, Korchnoi's defection notwithstanding.

♦ In 1982, PhysicsDude (my best friend at the time) got into *Star Trek*, which we watched regularly at his place with our peer group, and a part of that was seeing himself as Spock and me as Kirk, with chess an extension of our different personalities. He had read a few opening books, which influenced my play, though when he played the *Jerome Gambit*, a highly aggressive, equally unsound two-piece sacrifice, I lost interest. A few years later, when I had proper training and flipped our results, chess went from an important measure of intellect to a colossal waste of time.

♦ In August, 1982, a fellow street vendor and self-asserted strong player, refused to play me, because he had just drawn an international master (IM), and playing against me would have been too much of a letdown.

By 1984, I had a reasonably strong game, maybe 1400-1500 in strength, when I finally got in gear.

<u>Richard Gilmartin</u>

After a half-hearted suicide attempt and subsequent convalescence, I fell into a daily routine that had me awakening just after midnight, skating laps around the upper east side for exercise, and to just observe the nightlife, followed by the incredible quiet at dawn, after which I'd come home, nap, and head down to Washington Square Park on my bicycle. As I mentioned earlier, we'd trade his chess knowledge for my weed and a pizza for lunch, an absolute bargain compared to what most elite coaches charged, some up to $100.00 an hour. This was also during the first Karpov-Kasparov match, of which Gilmartin said *"the only time they look weak is when they play each other,"* which applied even more to the Williams Sisters in tennis many years later.

Gilmartin's lessons were brutal: if I didn't resign when lost, he would terminate the lesson, which caused me to study openings intensely, inadvertently taking Fischer's advice to devour *Modern Chess Openings* from cover to cover, which I did, amazed at how the book took for granted that I'd know why a move had an *exclam* (!), even if I remained baffled. By the end of the summer, I was tournament strength, thought to be Class B (1600-1800). After that came college, Kate giving me the score to *Chess*, and then the game taking a backseat once again due to the racetrack, where I was already winning money and threatening to win a lot more. I wouldn't do anything more until late 1986.

<u>**What I Do When There Is Nothing Else To Do**</u>

After I moved to Philadelphia in 1986, my business crashed, and I went broke figuring I could beat the mid-Atlantic tracks, leaving me with a lot of time and very little money. After contemplating the universe while spending three hours under hypnosis in a flotation tank, I walked home on an unseasonably warm Sunday evening, stopping at a used bookstore, where I picked up five chess books to go with my library of MCO, *Basic Chess Endings*, and *500 Master Games Of Chess,* to cover all three phases of the game, after which I made a fifteen-year plan to become world champion, and to make chess a repository for all of my free time, since I'd need a regular income or jackpot to fund this:

- *The Chess Struggle In Practice*, by David Bronstein. This classic, first-person account of the 1953 Candidates Tournament took me through the mind of its second-place finisher, giving me insight into what it would take to compete at that level. Most of the games were King's Indians, which made it a quasi-specialty book.

- *The Principles Of Chess*, by James Mason. I had never heard of Mason, and the book wasn't memorable.

- *Chess Fundamentals,* by Jose Raul Capablanca. The legendary world champion shared his insights, particularly into the endgame, but I found the text an oversimplification and too generalized to be of use to my game.

- *The Complete Chess Course,* by Fred Reinfeld. This "classic" taught me more about Reinfeld than chess, since everyone had an opinion of this prolific author, whose reputation precedes him, for a good reason.

- *King Power In Chess,* by Edmar Mednis. By far the most underrated of the five, Mednis's out-of-the box approach to king safety, including flipping him into an action hero when the need arises, fit well with my penchant for castling queenside, thanks to Mom telling me the king moved to b1 and not c1, and now for not castling at all!

By 1991, I would own well over a hundred chess books, covering every area of the game, including:

- *ECO Vol. A-E.* This classic five-volume set, with twice-yearly updates in the *Informant* series, were the ultimate in opening theory and resources until the engines took over at a much lower price. With a classification system that most players memorize, and main lines running up to twenty moves, it went a long way towards revealing to me how Kasparov and Karpov could reel off fourteen perfect moves in the Seville variation of the Grunfeld Defense.

- *Rook Endings, Queen Endings, Pawn Endings, King And Pawn Endings, Rook v. Minor Piece Endings, Bishop Endings,* and a few other titles I probably forgot, all $19.95 each from a specialty publisher. These books were invaluable in developing my technique, i.e., ability to close out wins, hold draws, or even swindle the occasional opponent.

- *The Najdorf Sicilian*, *The Complete Pirc,* and *The Benoni for the Tournament Player,* by John Nunn. These were invaluable resources, with the Pirc book enabling me to crush IM Anatoly Volovich (2508) out of the opening, before losing on time. The Najdorf book extended the main lines past move twenty-five, and on the verge of a forced draw, while the Benoni book explored lines popularized by Fischer, and convinced me not to play the Benoni, though I wound up playing it in reversed lines as White, a tempo to the good.

- *The Winawer French* (David N.L. Levy), and *The Pelikan Sicilian* (Shveshnikov), were the best of a dozen specialty opening books by several authors. The Pelikan was cutting-edge, challenging the notion that the backward pawn on d6 was fatal, revealing a highly enriching body of opening theory I taught to the high school I coached in 1990 from an 0-3 start to a 5-5 finish, third place in the city, and a 9-1 win in a pair of matches over Washington to end the year, with the team's babysitter (a teacher who was their tournament coach) telling me I should have been there to see it. I had beaten their star player eighteen months earlier, and got the intellectually dishonest *openings don't matter* lecture. I had schooled these kids for three hours a day, after waking up mid-afternoon, and on my way to Garden State. Three of the kids were one car behind the SEPTA derailment that killed three during morning rush hour.

- *How To Open A Chessgame*, by Larry Evans. The former national champion GM, and *Chess Life* columnist who published my game against Volovich in the August 1990 *Reader's Showcase* feature, as a warning that the clock was taking over the game, compiled a book with chapters written by seven top players, all revealing how they approached the opening, a *round table* format which was excellent except for one thing: all of them had lost badly to Bobby Fischer, whose repertoire I copied to begin my career, figuring any move that is good enough for Bobby was good enough for me, yet by 1988 I had completely replaced his repertoire with my own. I did use his Exchange Ruy Lopez as a panic "tunnel" to avoid that mountain of theory in the World Open, as I did not have time to prepare.

- *Encyclopedia of Chess Middlegames*. ECM is the tactician's bible, containing 3,001 middlegame positions, many from actual games, and now downloadable into a chess engine for further analysis, including many positions thought to be wins or draws that were not. Sometimes, even today's engines can take several minutes before finding the correct move, an indication that humans had evolved chess theory a great deal even without their help.

- *Pawn Power In Chess*. While staying at Murph's, I found a copy of this underground classic, then out of print, and his reaction when I saw it told me all I needed to know. Murph didn't part with his copy, but *WaiterDude* had one, which I learned while staying with him after a Thursday action tournament at the Manhattan (to which I commuted a hundred miles), and since he was no longer playing he gave it to me.

- *Domination in 2,545 Endgame Studies*. Easily the best chess book ever written, Kasparyan's incredible studies of "domination" (one piece controlling another) teaches the reader how to literally make their opponent's pieces fall off the board.

By 1991, I had an expert's rating at my peak, that dipped to 1900 at the very end, after I had been hired by Sol and mentally quit (not before hustling a tired Texan out of $25.00 in an all-night session), but chess had served its purpose, with me evolving from an aspiring world champion and the hardest-working player in the United States since 1987 (which anyone can accomplish regardless of talent), who caught the eye of sapiosexual women, to *chess degenerate*, even though I was on track to reach 2650 and top ten in the world, which scared me even more. With computers possibly rendering the game obsolete, it made sense to put chess on hold until much later in life, when I could build my *tunnel*.

Understanding the implications of Kate's gift to me opened up a previously hidden world, particularly where gorgeous sapiosexuals (I called them *minddiggers* in *Outfoxing The Foxes*) treated us the way sorority sisters treated jocks. Though at the time I bought into the intellectual dishonesty of women who generally disparaged my lifestyle because I wasn't a high-earner whose resources they could plunder, the exceptions were as notable as the highlight film:

♦ The primary knock against what I was doing with chess was that I was wasting my best *earning* years on a board game, which would make me a poor marriage prospect, as if my mission in life were to give up everything I enjoyed and half my wealth just to get laid on unfavorable terms.

♦ In July, 1987, I lost the under-1400 section of the World Open with a score of 5½ out of eight, losing the last game to the Bird Opening (1. f4). Thirty years later, I would adopt the Horsefly defense (1…Nh6!), which would have won easily. This was six months after I had met Murph, and where I first met Murph's mentor…*Emory Tate*, father of Andrew Tate, a man who both indirectly and directly taught me the Tate Mindset, but for an era nowhere near as cutthroat as this one. Suffice it to say that Andrew's existence surprises me not at all.

♦ In September, 1987, on an Amtrak train to New York for a chess tournament, I learned what the *Joffrey Ballet* was, when one of its fine (and I mean *FINE*) students connected with me as a "fellow artist," as she aspired to be a prima ballerina, with our paths in life taking us out of the corporate world and onto that train, on which no "sexy" six-figure white-collar worker could be found, as they were stuck in their offices. The significance of this lifestyle choice and prioritization of my time portfolio would only become apparent after I began working for Sol.

♦ Also in September 1987, I met a "road family" that let me stay with them whenever I was playing. My friends younger sister (too young but not for long), gave what I call the *who the f**k is THAT!?* look, very briefly, indicating she had never met anyone like me and was redefining her type. Cozy nature of this arrangement aside, almost all of my time was spent at tournaments, with the house little more than a pitstop, after which I'd get a ride to the train station and head home. This was not the type of women or families I would have met without my time portfolio.

♦ In May, 1988, SHBDancer (see *Bettor Off Single* for the sordid tale) notices me studying chess at the desk, and *connects* (her term) with me over our shared artistry. She was with a neighbhor, a seventeen year-old actor with whom she survived ten days in his studio on sex and a single takeout pizza, after which she had me call her a cab from my lobby, highly impressed that I had remembered her name, and even more impressed when I left her a note in her *NYU Tisch* dorm lobby, saying "why don't you throw a stone and pick it up over by the chess tables. I might be playing." The note was there in case she was around on the Saturday I had gone up to play, not for the *two weeks* she *stalked* me at the tables, as she let me know when calling.

♦ Also in May, 1988, I drew Asa Hoffman (2556) in a tournament game with Black, on a hundred-mile trip and two hours of sleep, awakening at 2:00 a.m. In the evening quad, I drew a Marshall Attack from future hedge fund king Boaz Weinstein, who took down the London Whale in 2009 by outlasting him on the other side of his rogue trade. I realized just how much opening theory there was to master, and began formulating the tunnel, though my original plan was to build it around the scripted main lines that were popular in the day. In between, I met the young lady who let me sublet her rent-*controlled* apartment in Midwood, at $360.00 for the month, in addition to the $125.00 a month I was paying for an attic on Forty-First Street. I would ultimately reject a life with her by ignoring her last-minute request to stay.

- My chess *groupie* in Midwood showed tremendous interest in me, particularly my DNA and the chess ability I might pass on to my children. She returned briefly from her travels to deposit her incredibly gorgeous cousin in my living room, on a half-hour's notice, assuring me that the woman was "quality," and was she ever! I also caught up regularly with Boards, WaiterDude, and PhysicsDude, as well as my family, but ultimately returned to Philadelphia rather than take over the apartment at market rent, not knowing that legally I could have made it rent-stabilized. By then, I was too entrenched at the desk and already had cheap rent. This cost me SHBDancer, who returned to NYU just as I was returning to Philadelphia.

- Thanksgiving weekend, 1988 was when my time portfolio paid its first huge dividend. I began the National Chess Congress at 3-0, nuking my plans to take a half-point bye in the fourth round, when SHBDancer would be coming by to pick up the five-page paper I did for her as a favor, not charging her because I knew she wanted to hook up. I tried to be the ultimate alpha male and win the game in time to make it home to *connect*, but failed on both counts. In the paper, she mentioned that massages from dancers are unforgettable, which I already knew. In retrospect, I should have taken the half-point bye and had her join me on Sunday after hooking up that night.

- In July, 1989, I was *stalked* again, this time by an incredibly hot sixteen year-old (perfectly legal in Pennsylvania), who followed me down Chestnut Street one morning, even crossing the street to match my movements. Cornered, I let her catch up to me and took her out to breakfast. She was one of many "live" women, long before I had "game." Chess was what I would later call a *gimmick*, but a very powerful one for which I was ridiculed for early in my PUA days, but time has proven me right with *The Queen's Gambit*.

- In February, 1990, I played the game against IM Volovich (a former champion of Moscow), which served notice that I was improving, but which also told me I was a step behind where I wanted to be, and set in motion my decision to quit the game the next year. I had just finished *The Complete Pirc* and went to the tournament intending to make a splash, which I did, just not enough.

- On Saturday, June 9, 1990, I had the ultimate logistical nightmare when, just as Go and Go was taking the lead in the Belmont, the radio broadcast went silent as my Amtrak ride to the eleven-round, all-night *insanity* tournament at the Manhattan, where rating points are won and lost in droves, entered the Hudson. My $20.00 win bet on Go and Go, placed by CycleDude at the track, paid $17.00, for a nice score, but separate pools at Garden State Park ($30.60) and Philadelphia Park ($38.40) made this one very expensive chess trip, especially considering the dime or so I could have won by diverting the entry fee and trainfare to a larger wager.

After 1990, I had few chess highlights, and played sporadically through 2003, when I joined ICC and got paired twice against Nakamura, holding my own in the opening each time. Until 2015, when I got my eyesight back and it was apparent I might live a few more years, I began training seriously again. Inspired by George Foreman, I decided not to rush my progress, or cut corners, making the odds of success slim. Indeed, my six-year plan failed completely, as I have managed "only" a 2337 peak Lichess rating, which has shifted my focus to tidying up loose ends and getting as far as I can, both to kill time before I die, and to assist future generations in continuing my work, which is now all but assured thanks to my win over Tariq Yue, and the e-mail from Leon that said he was 1700 and defeated an IM in tournament play.

A single win over a lone prodigy usually means very little, but for me, on that day, in that situation, it was huge, dispelling two ***intellectually dishonest*** myths: that I would fall apart at slower time controls, and that online ratings don't translate into "real life." Given that I was barely 1800 over the board, and ***2300+*** on Lichess, my win over a rapidly improving nine year-old (who is now rated around 2075 and top-four for age ten) is less of a shock. It also enabled me to quit playing over the board, since I had proven what I needed to prove, eliminating the need for hundred-mile trips to the Mashall or forty-mile trips to Paoli, each of which I made as much to prove I could survive the trip, as to play the games. My 4-11-1 record since my return is nothing special, but my recent performances also include a 2-0 start in a three-round under-2000 at the Marshall, and a near-win in game three. Most of my future live tournaments will be at the World Open or National Chess Congress, if at all.

Some reflections on the modern chess world:

♦ In the 1980s, I was one of very few people who took chess as seriously as Fischer, if not the only one. Most players trained maybe four hours a day, and the United States Championship was won by an IM one year. Our best players were routinely thrashed on the international stage. Even Kasparov did not seem unbeatable, nor even as talented as Fischer. Fast-forward to 2024, and my competition is five generations stronger, in a global, billion-dollar ***e-sport*** more like golf or tennis, with so many good players that winning a single major tournament, or even just getting the GM title, is more difficult than winning the world championship was in the 1980s.

♦ Even if the world title still mattered, online chess was nonexistent in the 1980s, and not an option; All indications are I'd have rarely if ever played over the board if it were. It was a different, long-gone era compared to the booming industry that is modern chess, fueled by the sale of neverending, expensive courses which purport to help you improve. To counter this, I publish my training materials (PDF, CTG, and PGN) absolutely free, or for a small fee on Kindle if you want to use that medium. This enables me to maximize my audience and save people a lot of money while also helping them to improve their game, which is very fulfilling.

♦ Thanks to the internet, the pandemic, and ***The Queen's Gambit***, I no longer have the ***wizard*** status high-rated chessplayers took for granted. In the dark ages (the 1980s), I might be the only tournament player someone encountered, their connection to the chess world, with my word as absolute gospel, and my ability to dominate the coffeehouse circuit considerable social currency. Today, even my 2337 Lichess peak does not stand out, winning takes a backseat to sexuality and popularity, livestreaming, and the billionaire owners of chess-related companies. Schools regularly advertise for chess coaches, some rated as low as 1200, near the minimum rating, but now a thousand points higher than the lowest. I have learned to appreciate my place in the top two to four percent of online players in my niche, and that I am at my lifetime peak at fifty-seven.

As I said in passing to a prodigy who certainly wasn't impressed with my rating, nor should he have been, I'm just another fiftysomething Class-A (now B) player with some stories, just like dozens of other men my age who prove their vitality by giving prodigies all they can handle, playing our small part to sharpen their teeth and prepare them for high-level chess, occasionally pulling out a life-affirming win, as we climb the ranks not by improving, but by merely staying alive, with something to do until the day I die, and not just checkers in a nursing home, but games which are actually relevant to elite play.

Essay #4:
You Can't Beat The Races

I never chose to be a gambler, and by the time I was given the choice, I was already profitable, which meant **_not_** gambling was very expensive, a flipping of the compulsive-gambling script. My answer to the "money" question on the Gamblers Anonymous intake form – *have you ever had a bailout?* – is an emphatic no. Not only that, but betting has gotten me out of far more jams than it has ever gotten me into, and is now performed strictly on autopilot, with bots that use proven algorithms that give me a chance to take down a jackpot, while saving handicapping time so I can devote more of my final attention to chess.

The racetrack is both intellectually honest and dishonest, and once upon a time was a fascinating American melting pot, where socioeconomic status was checked at the door (sorta), and anyone who entered the gates with as little as $2.00 could exit a wealthy man. Ernest Havemann's *My $61,908.00 Ordeal* documented his win in the *Five-Ten* jackpot wager at Aqua Caliente, from a $96.00 ticket that got him no partners, but lots of lectures on not wasting his money. The reader lived vicariously through this college professor's tale of how six winners changed his life, noting that this is all he would be remembered for, and predicting that someone would scribble *"it was luck"* on his tombstone two days after it, along with the story, was planted.

Harness racing, particularly the races on Channel 9 at 11:30, was a favorite family ritual, the culmination of a Saturday which began at an arcade, either in Midtown or on Mott Street (which I frequented alone many times after he died, as it was a straight shot on the M-15), followed by a stop at *Papaya King*, while Dad conducted business, and sometimes a trip to the track, particularly if Yonkers was running, as Roosevelt was an hour away even by car. I still remember Dad taking a free route home all the way through Queens because he didn't have toll money. At the track, I lived like an adult, handicapping as well as anyone else in the building, and methodically sharpening my skills, all with parental approval and consternation from everyone else.

After Dad died in 1979, it was almost as if I had never bet horses, though I made a couple of aborted trips to the OTB, which I found a waste of time even if I hadn't been kicked out due to age. The *Summer of Twelve* had me exploring Manhattan on my bicycle while doing messenger work for Mom and saving her a fortune, even after I began getting paid by the package. I did have all-night poker games but this was also a carryover from Dad, plus I had the only apartment with a "cool" parent. I didn't like the volatility so I stopped hosting these games, which never led to much in the way of wins or losses. I did spend a lot of time playing outdoors sports, but very little chess, squandering my potential as I aged out of a world title trajectory, all before puberty!

The 1980 Belmont marked the beginning of my true "career" as a horseplayer, with Mom informing me how much I missed the track, and maybe I did, but I was fine in the ensuing year and change. The day itself was marred by rain, causing us to scramble for seats in the third-floor cafeteria, with muted sound on the television (and Mom concluding that Andy Beyer was an idiot drunk). Mom was definitely influenced by the 53-1 winner, and I found it odd that she suddenly wanted to bet horses, because she had never shown any interest in going with Dad, even if her sister owned a stakeswinner at Monmouth in 1967. I was not about to turn down free money, and have very fond memories of the trips, including shaving an hour off the commute by catching the LIRR at Woodside.

The 1981 Baseball Strike ended my hero worship of baseball players, and soon after, my season ticket, and then attendance at any games, while freeing up the ***Summer of Fourteen*** for an intensive horseplaying bootcamp with Banned4Life, my connection for placing bets all day rather than waiting for Mom's one or two trips during her breaks. We won money almost from the get-go, especially after Mom taught herself to handicap at my urging. My early teens were marked by many windfalls, and I never stopped going to Yonkers and Roosevelt, mostly because there was little else to do, but after Ideal du Gazeau in 1983, I stopped almost on a dime, not winning again until my back was up against the wall in 1986. From there, five more profitable years ensued, again with haters reminding me that no one could beat the races, until Beyer released the Kraken in 1992, eliminating my edge for six years.

In 1999, when I released ***How To Break Even At The Track,*** the sport was still relevant, rebates had not yet killed the recreational player, and I had easily my most profitable years, thanks to the proliferation of national simulcasting, too late for me to cash in on from 1986-1991, but a steady ***side hustle*** until the bottom fell out after the big winning streak in early 2009, leaving me a gambling orphan until sports betting was finally legalized in 2019, albeit with the pandemic delaying me. Finally, however, the deaths of Maple Leaf Mel and New York Thunder were simply too much to stomach, and I have not wagered since, nor will I ever again, since the game is not profitable due to rebates, a huge waste of time to handicap, and no longer relevant or necessary.

It is definitely time to ***#endhorseracing***, preferably during Fashion Week, at Royal Ascot, with the Grand National moved there, so we can end all three plus abolish the monarchy in the ultimate ***woke*** grand finale. Most in the sport care for their horses as well as they can, but the sport itself is toxic and no longer woven into the fabric of American leisure, nor are the deaths freak accidents, but instead the result of abuse, drugs, and unsound breeding designed to fill betting fields rather than advance the breed. Hopefully we will take the final steps to making this a reality, even if it means a large hit to my time portfolio, as I was looking forward to doing PAP sheets with all this time to kill. Instead, SPX options have assumed this role, with better payouts, larger pools, and no horses breaking down and ***dying*** while four lengths in front as they cruise to the wire.

My position is nothing new: I watched Ruffian die on national television in 1975, at age eight, but it was Timely Writer's demise in the 1982 Jockey Club Gold Cup that really hit hard, given all the horse had endured to satisfy his connections' desire to compete. Not long after my big winning streak, and when the inner dirt track had just been rebuilt and reopened, jockey Amado Credidio, Jr., a promising twenty-one year-old, was killed instantly when he collided in midair with another horse. A female jockey, who had just moved off the rail right before the accident, described the horrors on Facebook, her own promising career derailed by back injuries. Unlike the animals, humans know the risks, but this doesn't absolve the sport, particularly one that rebates computer whales while ignoring my own request to have one percent of my handle diverted to aftercare for injured riders.

In 1987, I kept eye contact with Sydney Underwood, one of the most beautiful women I had ever seen at the track, dressed elegantly in the winner's circle. She smiled briefly then moved on, and I pondered what life would be like with a jockey as my girlfriend; it turned out she lived right near the track, while I had to commute home on Friday night, and then return for an afternoon card the next day (followed by a nice weekend). I forgot about this brief, powerful connection until 1992, when she was paralyzed in an accident at a poorly-lit Atlantic City Race Course, which terrified me on my only visit there six years earlier to bet Manila in the United Nations Handicap. She retained enough mobility to become a trainer, eventually retired and got married, and still living life to the fullest when last I checked. We chatted for a while, but a rejection like that isn't easy to get over…she is remarkable for what she's endured.

Horseplaying came through for me in 1986, when temp agencies were ignoring me in favor of women fed to the ***Wolves of Wall Street,*** the future ***#metoo*** predators who literally stole millions of dollars in lost opportunity, plus any growth in my real estate or stock holdings, which became clear to me in 1998, when a woman my age (thirty-one) earned six figures, owned a quarter-million dollar condo with no mortgage, and had a retirement nest egg of a half-million dollars, all because wealthy men wanted to have sex with her. That I am supposed to just ***get over it*** and say nothing twists the knife, and explains why a winning horseplayer is a threat to any conformist. Women, on the other hand, can easily avoid the risk of ruin with those oh-so-sexy white-collar men with stable jobs and their own place to live, yet have no problem helping me spend my winnings if I show up without revealing their source.

Essay #5:
Let No Man Put Us Under

You (male), meet another man in a social setting, and the conversation turns to your jobs. Using a strategy I call ***hover and pounce*** ("orbiting" to the PUA community), he senses opportunity:

"I'm a ***clinical hypnotherapist***. I help people eliminate bad habits."

A simple enough reply, except:

- He's not a licensed psychologist;
- He has not taken medical boards; and, while I'm sure this doesn't matter…
- He's ***gay*** and wants to have sex with you.

The last part doesn't matter, right? Hypnosis, a persuasion art, is rife with intellectual dishonesty that preys on public ignorance and imputation of magical qualities on what is essentially a biological process our DNA decided was useful for our survival, for some reason or other that has never been made clear. Your concern that your gay male hypnotist, who has already loaded your conversation with embedded suggestions designed to whet your appetite, might have ulterior sexual motives just isn't possible, and you really have issues and need ***therapy*** if you disagree; after all, he ***is*** a therapist! Besides, you don't have to worry because…

All hypnosis is self-hypnosis! You can't be hypnotized into doing something you wouldn't normally do. (Like have major surgery without anesthesia).

Whether or not you agree with this claim, if it is in fact true, it means that women and children who claim to have been raped or molested by a hypnotist must be lying. Even if that weren't possible, the existence of the ***hypnofetish*** calls into serious question why high schools invite stage hypnotists to perform, particularly when several of the men they hire for this also participate actively in the adult/fetish community, with some of their stray subjects wandering into our mature-themed chats before we sent them on their way with an advisory. I've often swayed concerned parents by asking them if they want me performing at their ninth-grade daughter's junior prom, noting that I could have easily done that, but won't do stage shows or therapy due to a conflict that too many ignore.

In recent years, the fetish has gone mainstream through hypnosis's redneck cousin, ASMR, with many women pulling down six-figure incomes on their video channels with titles like ***"Crazy Barber Kidnaps You And Gives Cranial Massage"*** On ***Brockmire***, the titular character referred to his ASMR video as "seducing a curtain."

Essay #6:
How To Pick Up Girls (The PUA Community)

When I was twelve, the earth moved, shaking my world view to the core. NBC ran a movie of the week about Eric Weber, whose self-published, bestselling *How To Pick Up Girls* (1970) made him a small fortune, and inspired a generation of hormone-driven tweens by showing it was possible to make money *and* get laid. "Dating expert" became a viable career path, one which would materialize two decades later, as we reached an age where those of us who were *Bettor Off Single* remained on the market, acquiring a decade or more of knowledge about women, knowledge which then began flooding the internet in the mid-1990s, first on *Netgirl*, as mentioned earlier, but then USENET, the platform that became a refuge for the male point of view, censored by AOL and Prodigy as "misogynistic." Like cancer, the truth metastasized into a *community* of pickup artists (#pua) who changed the world.

The highlight film from 1970-1995 includes:

- The *How To Pick Up Girls* movie, which mainstreamed Weber, the first PUA guru, who wrote his book after interviewing women on the street about what they liked in men. The most telling scene had Weber staring at an empty post-office box all week until a single slip of paper appeared on Friday, directing him to pick up two mailbags full of checks at the mail desk. The men who would go on to seed *#pua* with its powerful theory can almost all trace their origins to this landmark film.

- From 1981-1984, my cousin hooked up with Diane Lane, who turned up at Thanksgiving dinner in 1982 at his apartment. The best lesson from this interaction was that I remained after the meal with my cousins to watch football on television, while he took off with Diane. I heeded this lesson, always making sure to go out during the biggest sporting events, where I never found a shortage of sports widows eager to interact. Now that the NFL markets to women, this method is not as effective, though it still holds sway. It was only when I began advising others that I realized how above-average my own results were, since they didn't hold a candle to what he could pull off.

- *Nice Guys Sleep Alone* (1986). Bruce Feirstein's classic followup to ***Real Men Don't Eat Quiche*** (1982) was the wakeup call every nice guy needed, and the inspiration for *29 Reasons Not To Be A Nice Guy* (1999), my slap in the face to the *AFC* (Average Frustrated Chump). Back then, men shared war stories with other men, usually resulting in bad advice spreading, but when Boards and I did this, theory like the *pivot* evolved, after I saw the impact of "Lunch," a woman who later appeared in Playboy and who Boards would let leave the dining hall, then linger, as hot chicks would approach him. Even *Seinfeld* made a reference to this when George noted that one hot girlfriend was like a hand-stamp that let men come and go as they please into their "secret city."

- *Black And Single* (1992). Larry E. Davis's bestseller brought SMV to the masses, in a book I consumed during my lunch hours at UPenn.

- *Searching For Courtship* (1992). Winifred B. Culter, the author, called me in response to a letter I had sent her and liked my analogy that men play half-court defense with women, letting them make easy progress at first, while women play a full-court press. Her book filled a dating-advice gap by focusing on the supposedly lost but timeless art of courtship. As one who courts women he likes, I identified strongly with her world view, though her friendship with my bosses reflected our different circles.

- ***Men Are From Mars/Women Are From Venus*** (1992). John Gray's bestseller attempted to frame men and women as different alien species, but they aren't. Gray turned this into an industry that faded a bit into the background as the PUA community took over.

- ***Secrets of Seduction*** (1993). Brenda Venus, best known for her relationship with an aging Henry Miller, checks in with her taken on seduction, with stories of men she admired, including Steven Seagal, who she noted could take over a room even without fame because of how confidently he carried himself. A valuable text from the female point of view.

- ***Are You The One For Me?*** (1993). Barbara DeAngelis's extensive treatise on gender bias, and how men's economic oppression of women forces them to compensate by marrying their oppressors is a great read. She was the only author who eschewed advice on how to conduct a relationship with the far more important question of whether or not you chose the right person, noting that women should only date men they would want their children to be like. Awesome advice that is still way ahead of its time, and a strong influence on my own work.

At this point, I quit working corporate jobs except for the two law firms in 1994, and stopped spending my lunch hours in bookstores, except to read books on many topics. By then I was attempting to publish my own weight-loss book, a commentary on ***#prettyprivilege***, but was rejected by the six literary agents to whom I sent the book. In an interesting example of stereotyping, smaller publishers began offering to read my manuscript solely because I had registered my copyrights, an indication to them that I took myself seriously as an author. I did not send the manuscript out, because I wanted a big outfit to take it, instead shelving it for PowerBase, PAP (horses), and the internet message boards, which quickly dominated the landscape, on the way to dominating the industry.

While I used dating advice as a ***gimmick*** to attract women, and as a platform for my political views on gender bias, my extensive participation on Prodigy and AOL, and later USENET, was initially just a means of killing time that mushroomed into a lucrative business. In 1996, I connected with the future ***Anonymistress***, a hypno "switch" with whom I would take turns hypnotizing and being hypnotized by her, a rare experience even after all the hypnofreaks connected online, many of whom began selling audio, and later video, though my generation aged out of that market. I actually paid "Anon" $125.00 to record a free mp3 that raised the bar for free content, correctly surmising that the free samples from rival hypnodommes would follow suit, saving me a lot of money before I made even more with ***Hellen I and II***, a pair of audio mp3s.

Just as the internet became a dating-advice conduit, I was having my best results ever with women, particularly from 1994-1996, when I went from using chess to passively attract sapiosexuals, to someone who could make things happen from scratch, just by identifying women I knew were approachable and would be interested. Moreover, I didn't have to hit on them because merely ***talking*** to them meant they could continue the conversation if they became my girlfriend, simply as a result of mistake-avoidance and behavior congruent with that of a good boyfriend. Just ignoring them was enough rejection to ensure progress if they stayed, and time saved if they didn't. In a world of clueless men who were often virgins, or ***#incel*** (a term not used until 2009), my "game" seemed hall-of-fame material by comparison. By late 1996, I had more or less retired at my peak, content to kibitz in the "games" of others while sharing my method, eschewing relationships for the occasional hookup.

The First Pivot (1996)

In April, 1996, I received an e-mail from a young man who lived in the area, was stuck in the ***#friendzone*** by a woman he claimed to love, and was about to spill his guts the next time they went out to a bar, where his presence discouraged unwanted suitors (other than him). He asked my advice on what to say to her, and my answer surprised him:

"Stand her up."

"What? She won't want me if I do that!"

"She already doesn't want you."

"Good point. Won't she be mad?"

"Yes, but she'll never admit it."

"Why?"

"She'll call you Monday or Tuesday. Tell her you met a gorgeous woman at a stoplight and wound up having sex with her in a hotel, then add that she's such a good <u>friend</u> you knew she'd understand."

"You're demented."

"Your point?"

"What do I do next week?"

"Treat her like she's your cousin from any state other than Kentucky."

He did, and she melted, eventually hooking him up with six professional cheerleaders for local teams, an invitation I declined because I already had my own harem. This, of course, was at age twenty-nine, at the peak of my desirability, when I was in top shape, and most of my competition my age or older was married, divorced, had kids, or a nest egg and little else, plus no time, while younger men bored them to death, didn't understand them, and **couldn't sustain a conversation for more than five minutes** without losing their IQ to biology, and without her getting bored. At fifty-four, my last two girlfriends were nineteen and twenty, mostly because they liked long conversations, something any man can provide. It certainly wasn't what little was left of my looks or money.

My books disrupted the status quo on ASF, which some said was off-topic, but lots of PUAs moved in: me, Mystery, and a dozen or so other guys, including a television writer for a variety show whose identity I confirmed. Apparently, a parody of me showed up on television where I sued a nine-year-old for defamation and won **a***hole of the universe,** before being taken away in a spaceship. This was around the time when my haters weren't calling me a pedophile, that they were plagiarizing and pirating my work without even knowing it was mine. I was **cancelled** from ASF and the "community" long before it became cultural. The result of the censorship was that my materials became free to preserve my audience (I had books on other topics and betting plus below-the-line publishing support to pay my bills, plus the psych transcription gig).

The ASF FAQ

The short version was this:

"Because of trolls, ASF has moved to the ***moderated website,*** where Ray or any mention of his books is banned for trolling. If you must post here, here's how you can block him. Ray ***lives with his mother at thirty-four*** and suffers from mental illness."

Then, an automated post from a litigation-proof anonymous remailer would give Section 230 anyone who linked to it:

"More information about him can be found at ***harassthem.com*** or by doing a search."

This was back in the day when a ***serious tone*** and a diatribe of hate was all that was needed to be taken seriously. The "FAQ Administrator," who called my mother an ex-hooker and me a pedophile, was convicted of possession of child pornography in 2011, serving seventy-two months. Many on ASF actually turned to him for advice on Speed Seduction, and I was not the only one he attacked, at least before everyone but me made peace and build an NNTP forum designed to mimic ASF and newsgroups, no easy task at the time.

The commercial site controlled a large amount of traffic and only allowed certain advertisers, but faded with the rise of Neil Strauss, ***The Game*** (2005), and ***VH-1's The Pickup Artist*** (2007), along with ***Mystery's Lounge***, an invitation-only, "elite" underground site that bailed on ASF in 2000, to give live bootcamps, ***Real Social Dynamics*** (RSD), who cultivated a built-in pipeline for expensive bootcamps through city-based "lair" meetup groups, and ***Thundercat's Lounge***, which at one point had connections to prominent PUAs.

By 2009, the community collapsed under its own weight, but continued on with a new generation of ***#mgtow, #pua,*** and other new players, with George Sodini's killing spree in LA Fitness in Pittsburgh sparking feminist backlash that intensified with one notorious PUA making the cover of ***Time*** for being banned from several countries, this shortly after Elliot Rodger's killing spree in California on May 25, 2014, the evening I awoke to find myself once again public enemy #1 on twitter, but I wound up censored after complaining about being doxed and harassed, including with death threats, and with the inability to refute claims that conservatives were not being censored (I am generally considered ***anti-feminist*** though I would argue otherwise; Mom's brand of feminism was based on achievement).

The Rise Of Andrew Tate and…Pearl!?? (2014-present)

Around 2014, influencers like Andrew Tate took over where the rest of us left off, with a more hardcore approach similar to his father's chess training, which was intense, like the night ***Mate By Force*** (his team of hustlers that included Murph) had commandeered my bedroom at 1:30 a.m., turning it into an impromptu chess club consisting of the only five people in Philadelphia you could call at that hour (or after 10:00 p.m.) if you wanted a game against an 1800+ opponent, back in the ***dark ages*** of chess, when chess groupies stalked Class A players in Washington Square Park because they hadn't been schooled on how weak he was.

Andrew Tate rose to prominence because he made it easier for ***#incels*** seeking alpha isolation and improvement in life to talk to him than to talk to women, the same dynamic that gave rise to the ***Class of 1998*** on USENET, but, like chess, which is now several generations of young men removed from the low-hanging fruit (where the ***pivot*** could and did get any man laid), to ***#metoo*** and the feminist backlash that led to a global movement to "stop" Andrew Tate, as if that wouldn't just yield another replacement…enter ***Pearl***. ***Pearl***, who has already achieved one-name status, is a ***cancel-proof,*** British volleyball player from a wealthy family who says pretty much the same things as Tate, except she can't be attacked as a ***bitter, whining incel who can't get laid***, nor does she have a harem of webcam performers creating controversy, which makes her very difficult to attack.

Who's Lying?

The rise of Tate, Pearl, and the ***tradcon*** (traditional conservative movement) is the feminine equivalent of the male feminist, who exploits a vacuum by taking the "other" side in the gender war, almost the opposite of what John Gray did in the 1990s, this time without the ability to control the narrative that defined the ***pre-Game*** era. There are still 1990s-style gurus out there spitting out old theory, showing our work on USENET was not wasted, indeed setting the table for now, specifically because the fundamental question of who is lying – the nice guys, who say women want jerks, and the women, who say they make well-intentioned mistakes – was not answered in 2003, because I was not the voice of the "community," and even if I were, Hurricane Katrina wiped out most of Neil Strauss's appearances on the talk-show circuit, buying time before PUA truly mainstreamed with the VH-1 show, and of course with SNL doing a skit in 2008 where Bill Clinton wore a ***Mystery costume*** for Halloween.

All of the issues people deal with now: exclusion, deplatforming, censorship, and astroturfing, to name a few, were born in the 1990s, in places like USENET and on AOL, when the internet was truly up for grabs and ***billions*** of dollars were at stake. When I sued Google for ***$10 billion*** in 2004, that was my estimate of the damages caused by search engines that were swallowing content whole. In light of the trillion-dollar values of these companies, that amount no longer seems significant, yet I was ridiculed for this, by a small group of people trying to give the impression that the entire internet was up in arms; they weren't. Anytime you see an article that says ***People are…*** replace that with ***The author of this article <u>wishes</u> people were…*** our knee-jerk reaction allows the media to set trends because we assume they have fact-checked that people really are doing something ***en masse***.

Essay #7:
#defundwomen

Inevitably, by force of financial crisis, rather than boycott, reality will assert itself:

Men can live forever without sex; how long can women live without money?

The ***woke*** crowd's desire to see police and other perceived evils defunded inspired the recent trend where ***people are…***not doing anything different, but I wish more men were not spending money on women, which is actually true, but far short of the full-fledged ***boycott*** that would put the financial fear of God back into "romance." As of now, the ***#incel*** is funding his own demise by flooding money to women with whom he is not having sex, women who it seems never would have had sex as often as they did but for needing money. A return to those days is quite possible, but just as unlikely, because ***most money men spend on women for sex is not their own***, but corporate money in the form of ***#prettyprivileged*** hiring for anywhere from \$25,000.00-***\$25 million*** a year, money that also jacks up the price of stripclubs, prostitutes, and any ***#sexwork***, while also decreasing product quality, as the best women wind up ***stealth-whoring*** in corporate America. Face it: ***women have price tags***.

While my own prime years are testimony that money is not necessary to get the women you want, it definitely greases the wheels, improving logistics even if she is not profiting directly from your largess. The problem is not that a man must spend money to get laid, but with the total lack of value this traditional exchange now has, which is almost zero for the male, all because he is competing against nearly-infinite wealth, men who can "spend" money at no cost: an extra bedroom in their Park Avenue penthouse, a free seat on their private jet, or space in their tax-deductible Super Bowl luxury box, where she can network among the elite or one percent, a group with whom you can be sure she doesn't play games, or hard-to-get. There are ways to defeat these men and still get the girl, but most involve deploying, and thus depleting, extra time that you have and they do not, but when they do have time, they are making money while hanging out, while you are not.

The Spitzer And The Wealth Gap

In 2009, former New York governor Elliott Spitzer resigned amid a "scandal" that had him paying his own money for elite prostitutes, about 9-9.5 on the looks scale. The price of \$1,500.00 an hour that he paid was way up from the \$110.00 an hour I was quoted in 1981 by a service that advertised on ***Channel J***, the "porn superhighway" of Manhattan, inspiring me to call a ***Spitzer*** the amount of money it takes to have sex with the hottest (and most skilled) prostitutes, as an economic indicator. Today, that price is \$5,000.00 up to ***\$25,000.00 a night***, and worth every cent, as this is what the sexual marketplace will bear. The sharp increase in the value of a ***Spitzer*** is tied directly to the wealth gap, where a decreasing number of wealthy men outbid each other, all of whom have money to burn.

At the end of the day, wealthy men are trading what to them is ***toilet paper***, and to most men a month's income or more, for some of the best sex the planet has to offer. Still, I will not patronize prostitutes at any price, though I will and have accepted freebies, including the night I lost my virginity to a \$2,500.00-a-night callgirl (up to about \$200.00 an hour from 1981) because some geezer was too depressed over Gary Hart losing to go through with his date. I consider prostitution to be ***bought rape***, since money is the only reason she wants the sex. There are actually prostitutes in Canada who give freebies to homeless men as if they would food, and bless their souls, but I cannot look forward to or have great memories of sex with any hooker, plus she might be trafficked or abused.

I will tip a stripper generously or give gifts like expensive jewelry (quicker than talking), which they can "wear or sell," and if she wants to have sex later, that's fine but it's not required (this avoids making it a trick). Stripclubs are a gray area that I also generally reject due to lifestyle and privacy issues, particularly on the internet, which makes any relationship akin to junior high school, with the potential for gossip. The other problem is that women who used to strip or turn tricks now set up websites and make six figures without ever having to interact. I did shop for prostitutes recently and the one I wanted cost $5,000.00 a night, if I went that route. These prices have caused me to alter my betting and trading accordingly, as I am to win *stripper money* rather than just a few extra bucks, but the times I have won that much, I've not purchased any sexwork. By the same token, I spent very little on my last two girlfriends, but they were costing me too much time.

The Free-Money Gambling Date

In 1991, I dated a woman who refused a second date on the grounds that her parents wouldn't let her date a gambler, classic intellectual dishonesty, since she'd have broken any rule that suited her. The date was simple: I buy lunch, set aside $20.00 for betting, and she gets half of whatever is left at the end of the day, a great way to bond and maybe win some money. Our date wound up on a day where I won $575.00 and kept it all, though I didn't have a big score until the last race at Penn National, but I did win about $200.00 at Philadelphia Park. Had I just shown up with that money and never admitted to betting, I'd have made more progress; ironically, I was working for Sol while she was "finding herself" in a nicer apartment than mine, subsidized by her parents.

In April, 2023, I made a series of trips to an area stripclub, spending about $1,200.00 in five visits, mostly just to see if I could make the trip to NYC or Paoli for chess tournaments, which also involved travel and several hours at a venue. I budgeted a few hundred for each visit, which was very well-received, and I gave earrings to a few dancers. One dancer, however, rejected my gift of futures bets on the Knicks and Lakers to win the title, on the grounds they would lose. She was right, and the bets tripled in value, plus PowerBase is a futures monster, having just paid for these visits with Florida Atlantic at 40-1 to make the Final Four, with Barkley claiming anyone who had that bet was lying. I couldn't believe the dancer flat-out *rejected* not only my money, but free picks, and *hundreds of dollars in free money* as a new customer, with PowerBase able to supply enough picks to churn any bonus, a very lucrative offer that fell on deaf ears.

The Saturday prior to Week 13 of the 2023 NFL season (PowerBase was written for basketball so the day of the month in the date reflects the NFL week), I went back to the stripclub to see if any dancers wanted to spend Sunday at the club tapping into all the free betting money and using PowerBase's picks to churn the bonus money, for at least a few hundred dollars, completely risk-free, and a lot more if the bot had a good week. This would also be a way to bond with a good customer, but this is exactly what strippers do not want. As it turned out, this was the one week that dancers shouldn't have ignored the offer, though most weeks the results are not that extreme. Here, however, they were.

```
                       Slow    Fast                         Slow    Fast   Slow    Fast    Power
Time Power Favorite    Rating  Rating  Power Underdog        Rating  Rating Line    Line    Total   Open  400am Vegas3 Pick Stars
---- --------------    ------  ------  --------------        ------  ------ ------  ------  ------  ----  ----- ------ ---- -----

Games of Mon,  11/13/2023:

2015 DALLAS             99.95   99.56  Seattle               95.54   95.12   8.41    8.44   51.18   6.5    8.5  46.5    2    -2   41-35 (w)
1300 LA Chargers        93.49   94.09  NEW ENGLAND           86.50   85.49   2.99    4.60   47.25   3.5    6.0  40.5    1     5    6-0  (T)
1300 Detroit           100.46  100.52  NEW ORLEANS           93.24   93.33   3.22    3.19   44.20   2.5    4.5  45.5    1     4   33-28 (w)
1300 NY JETS            91.55   90.87  Atlanta               90.69   90.31   4.86    4.56   31.95  -1.5   -3.0  34.5    2    -8    8-13 (w)
1300 PITTSBURGH         99.07   99.84  Arizona               85.56   86.24  17.51   17.61   43.47   3.5    5.5  39.5    2   -10    3-17 (W)
1300 TENNESSEE          91.67   92.67  Indianapolis          94.04   94.58   1.63    2.10   44.85  -1.5   -2.0  42.5    2    -1   28-31 (w)
1300 Miami              99.75   98.93  WASHINGTON            90.48   88.14   5.27    6.79   69.48   7.0    9.5  49.5    0     0   45-15 (X)
1300 HOUSTON            96.20   96.44  Denver                95.28   95.04   4.92    5.40   55.24   3.0    3.5  46.5    1     2   22-17 (w)
1605 TAMPA BAY          90.86   91.24  Carolina              83.87   84.52  10.99   10.73   33.47   5.5    5.5  37.5    2    -7   21-18 (W)
1625 PHILADELPHIA      106.88  105.45  San Francisco        100.84  101.96  10.04    7.49   56.76   2.5   -2.5  46.5    2    -8   19-42 (w)
1625 Cleveland         100.07  101.94  LA RAMS               93.41   93.91   2.67    4.04   33.44  -1.0   -4.5  39.5    2    -4   19-36 (w)
2020 Kansas City       102.13  101.71  GREEN BAY             93.92   93.74   4.21    3.98   41.19   6.5    6.5  42.5    2    -3   19-27 (W)
2015 JACKSONVILLE      102.13  102.60  Cincinnati            96.22   96.21   9.90   10.39   37.23   7.5    7.5  38.5    2   -10   31-34 (W)
```

That's ***11-0-1***, a record I didn't even achieve, having gone "only" 8-0-1 (by eliminating the 1-2 star picks). Several of the games barely covered on last-minute scores in garbage time, but the fact remains that any stripper who had agreed to this "date" would have made ***tens of thousands of dollars*** on the round-robin parlays alone. Also note the moneyline winners with Green Bay and Cincinnati, which greatly amplified the parlay payoffs. A twelve-team round robin that pays on 11-1 or better costs all of $1.30 (including the twelve-teamer), and all twelve eleven-teamers would have hit. Now add hedging at the end, and the wide middles that opened up, and we literally would have broken the bank. This was the night ***#defundwomen*** was born, since they didn't value my brains, my knowledge, or my ability to connect them with free money, or in this case, a jackpot.

Women Are Financially DIFFICULT

Thanks to chess, I can attract even wealthy women if they are sapiosexual, but when money is involved, they will make themselves so logistically ***difficult*** that you'll be laying out money for the many unnecessary expenses they create, if you try to pursue them, or show up at their club with an offer worth five figures that they thumb their nose at because they'd rather grind someone for not even a hundred. Since this spending won't improve your chances of getting laid, saving your time and money is correct. If more men did this, the sexwork market would crash, or come back within the Spitzer's historical range, adjusted for inflation. Generally, if you're not budgeting five figures or more, and you don't know how to pick the right women, don't waste your money, especially if you're not getting laid, since you're also contributing to the massive spike in the ***#incel*** population, as women no longer need our money.

I no longer offer coaching, though my books still sell, indicating that they remain relevant within their niche, but I want no part of telling other people how to live their lives, though I am proud of my legacy and having altered the DNA pool in the only way I ever will, as I never had children (that I know of). I see a lot of intellectual dishonesty, mostly from people who either don't know what they're doing, who charge money, or a combination of the two. I'm glad that the truth has come out a great deal more now than in the 1990s, but the overall picture for the average men and women is bleaker than it's ever been. I suppose AI bots will become surrogate partners, but this is so…***synthetic***. It's also very lifelike and the market is already growing exponentially, even with relatively crude offerings.

Recently, Colin Cowherd devoted considerable airtime to Taylor Swift's haters, saying that you can tell a lot about someone by the little things that bother them, or something to that effect, ignoring that he was incredibly bothered by *"weird, lonely, insecure men,"* i.e., the stereotypical *#incel*. This tired narrative is based on the false premise that men are sex-addicted horndogs perpetually lusting after most any woman in sight, can't control themselves, and are the cause of women's *sexual paranoia,* as if women didn't encourage men to "wait for their soulmate" or promise that the "right woman is out there," encouraging them to "go for it" when they find one they like, but to "forget her and move on because she wasn't the one" if she doesn't, meaning his feelings don't matter. To avoid this verbal abuse, a man is encouraged to find the hottest chick who says yes, not the one he really wants, then women complain that their man "settled" for them by "marrying the girl in front of them."

Pretty Women Are The New White Men

Males have been relegated to the role held by women in the 1950s: be attractive, pleasant, don't make waves, and defer to women, if one wants to advance in life, in her case through marriage, and in his through not being cancelled. I gave up d/s (dominance and submission) in 1996 not because it wasn't working – my submissives loved the attention and guidance – but because anything I did could have been retconned as abusive; see my *NFL replay booth* analogy from earlier. This has expanded into a general aversion towards minimizing contact with others, since privacy is long gone, with any conflict having the potential to become the next internet drama into which one is involuntarily thrust. The mating game is still alive, of course, but has changed so drastically that it barely resembles what it was in my prime, and I am no longer dialed in socially, even if I can still land a stray girlfriend here or there.

Men who don't like the power women have are going to have to adapt, since nothing is going to change. Their sexuality, and the minor technicality that *women give birth* will always make them more important than men. I can be the biggest *alpha male* in the world but still have only the fraction of power that women enjoy just by breathing, with attractive women elevated to apex-predator status. Like a 1950s housewife, I can protest the injustice and oppression, or work within it to get ahead. What I can do is make myself attractive or useful to women, and that hasn't changed in the past thirty years. A man can always raise his SMV, as I recommended in *Foxes*, all the way through to *Bettor Off Single*. I do not envy young men today, as they are in a sexual dust bowl created by online patronage from simps that allows women to post a few PG-13 pictures and make six figures or more.

If you are going to use money to get laid, you need to outspend your rivals, and find the women who offer the best value, whether in a direct transaction, or within the pretext of a relationship. Sexwork is an option but like finding good barbecue in Georgia, or a good cheesesteak in Philadelphia: too many inferior products trading on general popularity without offering quality. Though the risk is reduced with the $5,000.00-a-night hookers, all bets are off on the internet, plus many of these workers screen their clients, an indicator of their lifestyle problems for which you have to pay with your privacy. Most men go for a "stealth" sexworker, i.e., a golddigger or a woman who finds high-earning men "sexy" while imputing nonexistent flaws on men like me rather than admit they just want money; this sounds benign but is why few men carve out the creative path I did, the one that pays much better in retirement than a nest egg, though I have little for a woman to plunder unless she wants a gambling date.

I lost my taste for using money with women when my attempts to make them large amounts of money fell on deaf ears, a rejection not just of me, but of the one thing I had to offer, that they weren't able to recognize, or simply didn't care if they did. I'm not going to pay through the nose for a woman who is just there to take the money and run, especially since treating it as "real work" with a negative review, negotiating price, or otherwise complaining is deemed harassment. If that's the proposition, I'll keep my money to myself until such leverage arises as in the financial crisis of 2008-2009. During my stripclub visits I realized that I did not get one dollar poorer just because some dancer didn't think I was worth her time, nor one IQ point dumber just because she didn't find what I had to say interesting or useful. By waiting for that "right woman," in this case one who values what I have to offer, I have saved myself a lot of grief that many men consider unavoidable.

As for your own love life, that's not my business, nor would I know what to tell you so many years after I was on much different playing field. Those who claim to are engaging in a very intrusive business where they claim to solve the most important aspect of your life, just as I did in 1998. It's not something I'd easily consider repeating were I given the chance, but that's how it went down.

Essay #8:
Money Management

Regardless of your age or situation, finances will dominate your life. Having grown up ridiculously privileged even if I wasn't a millionaire, with parents as brilliant and creative as they were well-off (amplifying the impact of their money), and physically gifted (dad was a champion swimmer and Mom could have been an athlete), and then having been trained to win money since toddlerhood, I have generally never obsessed over it, regardless of how much or little I had. My 1990s haters who pointed out that I *lived with Mom* and actually believed that to be a negative are giving the right answers to the wrong questions. We landed in Philadelphia in 1986 with barely the shirts on our backs, and rebuilt a nice life for the next few decades. I am now retired on a fixed income so my situation is rather normal; if I do break the bank, it'll be through chess or a jackpot win.

As I've already noted, nest eggs are nice, for as long as they last, but everyone should plan for the day where they have to live like me, on a fixed income that can be pretty high with a good pension or social security benefit, but even my modest benefits are enough for survival and even a decent lifestyle, though one where I have to watch every cent. That I can still win money betting or trading or make it writing and teaching chess, and that these skills are still profitable in old age, nor can they be seized in bankruptcy, while keeping me socially active and relevant (see the win over Tariq Yue), makes my *time portfolio* my most cherished asset, one that pays dividends every time I trade an option, make a bet, or play chess. I make money whenever I can, but also make sure that my time is never wasted, with chess as the repository for when I have nothing else to do.

Betting

I already published *The Fix Isn't In*, which documents PowerBase and PAP (for horse racing), and which is free through a link on my YouTube channel (in the video announcing the book), so I don't need to cover that here. Instead, I'll share my philosophy:

- ♦ I am a *jackpot hunter*, in that my primary goal is a life-changing score, which I have yet to fully achieve, though I have had many four- and a few five-figure windfalls that have provided me with up to six *Spitzers*, for those looking to convert their winnings into women. Usually when I win I pay down my credit cards, and pay as many bills as I can well in advance so that I have a cushion if things go sour, and so I'm not betting money that is already spent.

- ♦ I *detach* from my results, which is easy to do because my wagering is automated. Literally *bet it and forget it*, often checking scores once at the end of the night, and trusting my bots even if they pick teams I wouldn't. In the offseason, I review the previous season and finetune my angles accordingly. I also regularly make futures wagers, since PowerBase excels at finding the best teams

- ♦ I bet *only what I can afford to lose*, now a fixed amount per month, usually the few dollars I have left over after I pay my bills. The ability to *roll up* small amounts into large amounts is useful, since the sky is the limit with house money; indeed, you can play completely risk-free if you want, through bonus money and sponsored contests, and literally ***win your way up***. I once turned a spare $0.40 into $287.60 on a superfecta picked off the board at Beulah, and turned $0.70 into $960.00+ at Parx with a superfecta key and cold combination. From there anything is possible, especially if one does their handicapping. Thanks to my bots, I have no difficulty scaling up or down my wagers, and won't hesitate to stop betting or cash out a wager should the need arise.

- ***Total cash is all that matters***. I'd rather have a negative ROI and money in the bank than be profitable and have that eaten up by living expenses. This sometimes requires me to stop betting or cash out a future, but avoids the risk of ruin that can happen when one gets too greedy or aggressive due to perceived opportunity.

- ***Pick winners and the rest will take care of itself***. "Money management" is a sham concept, since it presumes an edge; acquiring that edge is key, though it requires a huge leap of faith and a lifetime of work (easy money is never easy because so many people chase it). In a world of intellectual dishonesty, it is easy for bettors to be misled, especially when those who reveal the truth are censored, and the audience fails to consider that they are being manipulated.

- ***Reduce your handicapping time***. Unless you have a job in the industry, like Beyer with horse racing, wasting time watching games and analyzing a mountain of statistics costs money that could be made doing other things. My chess rating is the product of all the time I saved by automating my betting and trading, plus it removes emotion from the game, while setting parameters for the results I can expect, though I never thought I'd go 11-0-1 on an NFL Sunday, even if I'd gone 1-14 a few years ago (and still had a winning record).

- ***Be a contrarian.*** Though not as powerful now as in the past, underdogs and under-the-total tend to do well, as does in-game bets on teams that are far behind (often +500 or more on champions facing elimination, like the 49ers against the Packers in 2024 or the Chiefs in several of their big wins from down twenty or more). At the track, many favorites are vulnerable to a strong challenger, while in the stock market, direction changes all the time as one narrative gives way to another, with the SPY moving 50-100 points in a few months in an unexpected direction, offering jackpot potential for those willing to bet options and buy or hold when everyone else is selling or vice versa.

In my ***final*** years, I have greatly toned down my betting and trading, mostly because I don't ***need*** money the way I used to. I am still a jackpot hunter, but take much more pleasure in a simple, predictable lifestyle that lets me focus my remaining energy on chess or other creative pursuits. If I get hot, or my bot locks in to a good bet, I will certainly capitalize, but my life no longer centers around wagering, because chess is too lucrative in ways money can't measure. As I have already said, I wouldn't trade my win over Tariq Yue for any amount of money, because the record of that game, and its relevance, is literally eternal, especially if he becomes a champion. Unfortunately, women focus so much on money that men follow their lead and downplay everything else.

Essay #9:
Let Me Be The First To Say...FAREWELL!

Though well aware of my mortality ever since my first poodle died on my terrace, like most, I detached from the reality that now confronts me perpetually, making every day potentially my last, while I know that as of now, based on laboratory testing, that I have a 1.9 percent chance of dying within the next three months, a 15 percent chance of dying within a year, and a 56 percent chance of dying within five years, way up from before I got my weight under control with a high-protein diet which may or may not help, but which certainly hasn't killed me. I do my best to take good care of my body, quit drinking in 2018, quit smoking in 2010, and avoid taking chances as much as possible, though I refuse to stop traveling to places like chess tournaments, stripclubs, or other venues. As I am increasingly fragile, I have to be much more careful with regard to things that would literally bounce off others, like extreme cold (I have thermoregulation issues), or bleeding (low platelets).

One area where my functionality has not diminished is chess, where I have somehow avoided recognition as an *adult improver*, despite an 837-point rise in my rating in the past nine years, on top of improvement of several hundred more points in my twenties, when even then I was considered washed up. If my progress doesn't prove that age is no impediment to improving at chess, I don't know what would. More pressing issues are *death*, which would stop my progress, as well as priority, in that most will have better things to do than train hard at chess, and even if they did, there is a law of diminishing returns, since dying with a 2400 or 2500 rating won't change much over my current legacy, though it will definitely improve my work for those who continue it, which is why I do it, and I can't say for certain even now that I won't achieve perfect play. Even if I "fail," I still have a great way to kill time that is not "checkers in a nursing home."

Turn It On Again (Brushes With Fame)

The *Genesis* song of the same name has the line "I can show you some of the people in my life." In a world where some meet only one or two celebrities in their entire life, usually in public or at their events, fame came crashing through my door early and often, not only demystifying celebrity, but introducing me to its downside, no more so than watching my friends and relatives turn into my *parents*, warning me of severe consequences if I leave a negative impression on people about whom I did not give a flying fuck. It also annoyed me that the moment the celebrity was gone they would revert to actually caring about me, something they shouldn't have suspended along with their brain. These betrayals would inevitably lead me to terminate the friendship, a bit down the road to mask this reason, since anyone who attempts to assert *parental* authority over me loses the privilege of interacting with me, with no second chances.

The highlight film here is incomplete, as I cannot remember every famous person who has ever crossed my path, but I'll do my best:

- *Gordon McLendon*. While I was not named after the legendary Texas businessman, I did get my middle name (Roy) from a *business deal* involving McClendon, while my first name was my mother's maiden name. Unfortunately, Roy Lofton (the other part of this deal) would never have believed this, so I was given his name for my middle name. On the internet, I changed my name to Ray Gordon to honor my mother, who put me through private school after Dad left us with nothing but a pile of bills when he died. Mom even wound up surpassing him as a horseplayer.

- ***"Lucky Pierre" Salinger***. JFK's press secretary's first newspaper job was picking horses, hence the nickname. He and Dad were so close that Dad was his only outside contact when Pierre went undercover as a prison inmate, and for a brief spell in 1976, my living room became Jimmy Carter's New York City satellite headquarters, replete with all-night poker games. I used to have a scanned dinner-party picture with Pierre seated next to my much younger and extremely hotter parents, circa 1966, that would have been included here were it not lost.

- ***William "Bill" Goldman*** and ***Arthur Ashe***. Each were Mom's longterm clients, and I once awoke with Goldman standing over me in my living room while I was sleeping on the couch, admiring Mom for tending to me. Ashe lived a few blocks away, which is why he called us, and I would pick up or deliver work from the lobby of his building.

- ***Anthony Mirra and the "DiMAYO Brothers."*** Thanks to YouTube channels like the very popular Sammy "The Bull" Gravano's "our thing" podcast, I learned more about my apparently mobbed-up family than I cared to, particularly Tom and Roy ***DeMeo***, as well as legendary mafioso Anthony Mirra, Mom's boyfriend while estranged from Dad (into her office that was our dining room, but back into his bed before he died), who I interrogated in the building driveway, asking how he knew Mom ("friends"), and what he did for a living ("business"). He couldn't have been more polite, and contrary to other accounts, was never abusive. Not sure if Dad knew about him but he'd have had no more fear than I did. I guess Mirra liked that I was looking out for Mom; he was whacked in January, 1982, which I learned from the front page of the ***New York Daily News***.

- ***Howard Cosell and Jimmy The Greek***. In 1978, I sat down at a coffee shop next to ***The Mouth That Roared,*** and roared it did, when I asked his opinion of the Mets and the Seaver trade, and the Jets and Giants. He could have made reciting the menu sound fascinating, and was pretty much what I expected. In October, 1980, I ran into ***The Greek*** outside the dining room at Belmont, asked him about his pick of the Jets to win the Super Bowl, and he said simply "I was wrong." I also won $30.00 on a 6-1 shot I went onto over the 8-5 favorite I overheard the legend wager $200.00 on to win, my first true contrarian play.

- ***Burt Young***. In December, 1981, I was skating down Lexington Avenue, when ***Paulie*** from the Rocky movies calls me out: ***"Look at the kid on the skates!"*** I stopped, skated up to him, and shook his hand and said "Hey, you're ***Burt Young!***" No doubt he was impressed I knew his name, thanks to my habit of watching the credits after each film, and HBO showing ***Rocky*** twenty-three times in February, 1978, my first month with the service.

- ***Michael "Momma Walton" Learned***. The four-time Emmy winner married my half-brother in 1979, with my first alcoholic beverage consumed on the double-decker bus to the reception at the Waldorf-Astoria, where I met my twenty-six year-old "half step nephew."

- ***Michael Rapaport***. Our mothers were friends, so we had to be nice to each other, and got along well enough without really being close, though we spent time in each other's apartments. Michael was such a quiet child, always respectful and polite, never even cursed, and grew into the fine man everyone knows today, who offends absolutely no one.

- ***Rodney Dangerfield***. On second thought, perhaps Mom should have moved us into his ***four-bedroom***, rent-stabilized apartment on a higher floor in our wing of the building in which we were neighbors, where he routinely hit on her in the elevator, and where I'd often run into his daughter (now a designer) in the elevator while, especially when we were walking our dogs (I mostly used the stairs otherwise).

♦ ***Cynthia Nixon***. My grade-school classmate called me out in front of the arcade that would close after a murder in 1984 (where they were looking for someone who looked like me before killing an innocent, just as I had stepped out), one afternoon in 1982. It was a definite ***Sex And The City*** moment, though we were pulled apart by our annoyed friends after ten minutes or so, just as I was getting ready to ask for her number. Since she couldn't have me, she did the only logical thing and became a flaming homosexual, whose campaign slogan for Governor was ***Vote for the homo, not for Cuomo***, flipping the latter's father's whisper slogan from 1977.

♦ ***Steven "Young Sheldon" Molaro***. After spending the summer of 1982 goofing around on the telephone, and meeting at my vending cart, we parted ways, with him returning to sixth grade in Whitestone, and me beginning my junior year at the next guest's high school. I looked him up a few years ago and found he created a television show and character with whom you might be familiar. He was not famous when I knew him, though his career certainly didn't shock me. He ***was*** Young Sheldon pretty much, just as curious. His bedroom is also where I saw my first personal computer: his ***Apple II***. He was very advanced for his age and for that era. His success is no surprise.

♦ ***Diane Lane***. My cousin's ex-girlfriend from high school. I shared a holiday meal with her. I did not hang out much with them except at funerals or weddings. Diane knows a lot more about what's going on with that side of my family than I do, which I find amusing. She was very polite, civilized, and since everyone walks on eggs around celebrities, nothing noteworthy happened except her and my cousin disappearing for the NFL games I watched with my other cousins, while gorgeous women everywhere languished. So clueless was I at the time that I didn't think to invite a struggling actress who was renting a room from PhysicsDude to meet them.

♦ ***"Mystery."*** As business rivals who found the same incubation pod in 1998, we got to know each other, but were not friends, and I rejected his offer to "wing" with him back when he was building his name. His influence on the ***#pua*** community is well-documented, while mine was more under the radar, as I did not go mainstream, and ***#pua*** was a small part of my focus on multiple topics of general interest to men, particularly betting. This allowed me to survive without the need to turn a profit in this niche, though I certainly have and continue to make the occasional sale of a book written decades ago.

♦ ***John Doe***. A very famous Hollywood writer who probably would rather remain anonymous used to contribute selections for the California Tracks to ***United Free Handicappers*** before I shut it down. We would chat from time to time.

My childhood made me celebrity-averse for the most part, since they are spread too thin to spend significant time with, plus I have my own life. I mention these people because the readers are familiar with them, and in most cases, I didn't just know them, but they know me, mostly on a surface level but certainly not at a meet-and-greet. They are not normal people but they know how to behave in public and private, and most tend to be driven, which is how they became famous. Perhaps when I die they'll take a moment to share, but I'm not holding my breath, and won't be then. I did not include ***public figures*** on this list, limiting to mostly A-listers that I didn't seek out, and that one of my peers that I happened to be close with turned out to be an A-lister suggests that my lifestyle and geography played a role.

I don't dwell at all on death, beyond preparing for it as best I can, while preserving my remaining functionality. I have no real complaints, particularly as I watch most or all traces of me and my work fade into the background. What seems so intense at the time rarely remains that way as time marches on and the world changes into something I barely recognize compared to my youth, when the *safe space* was your school's nuclear *Fallout Shelter* in the basement, and hurt feelings were a fatal weakness in dealing with life's adversity. Shows like *Cobra Kai* explore this dynamic through Johnny Lawrence, a throwback to a long gone era before political correctness.

I've taken great pains to preserve my work for those who wish to continue it, and making it freely available to maximize its reach and eliminate any cost barrier, while I continue to put the finishing touches on chess. I'll be streaming a lot more once my rating clears another level or two; no one really cares until someone reaches the top and is clearly on the way. All indications are the *tunnel* method is increasing in popularity, particularly with a 1700-rated player defeating an IM, or so he claimed in an e-mail to me. Having *something to do* every day is nice, though even if that were just binge-watching shows I missed in the 1990s, like *Frasier*, that would be fine as well (I've done that for days or weeks at a time as well).

My retirement began early and will end early, probably very uneventfully, at which point the internet will take note, life will go on, and my work will be mentioned from time to time, hopefully without all the temporal garbage attached. Namecalling isn't much of a legacy.

I have added the *tunnel* chess book as an appendix, in case the other links disappear from the internet after I'm gone. It is also available separately on Kindle.

The TUNNEL:
Forcing (At Least) A Draw From Move One

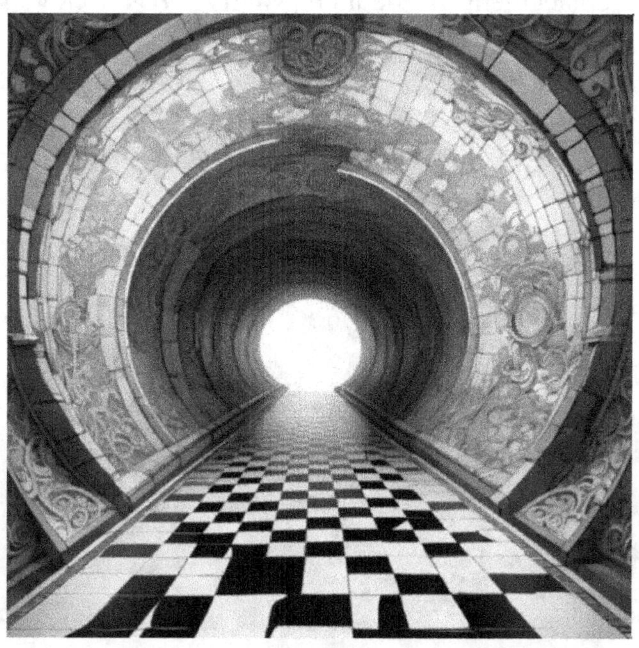

By RAY CHARLES GORDON

***Cover Image created with Canva's AI image generator (https://wwww.canva.com)**

Foreword

Bill Bastable chose videogames over chess. Having met him and seen him play PacMan, and having seen Bobby Fischer's chessgames, the better gamer of the two is very clear. HINT: it's not Fischer.

This is 9x9 chess, a replacement for the increasingly *solved* 8x8 version:

The Official Rules Of Ray Gordon 9x9 Chess (RG-99)

I. **The Board**

RG-99 is played on a 9x9 board, with eighty-one squares with coordinates a1-i9, as below:

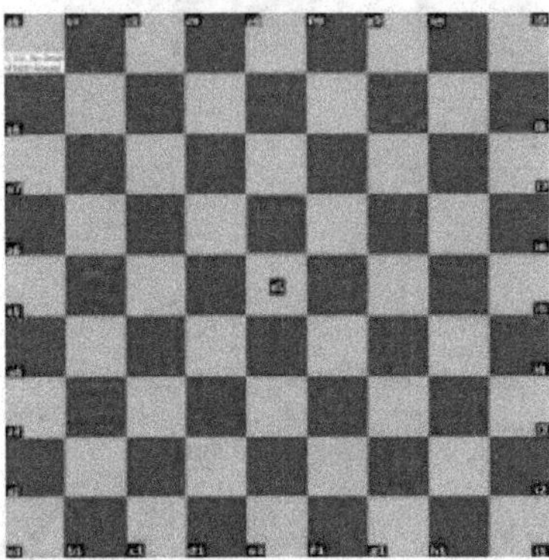

The pieces are set up as follows:

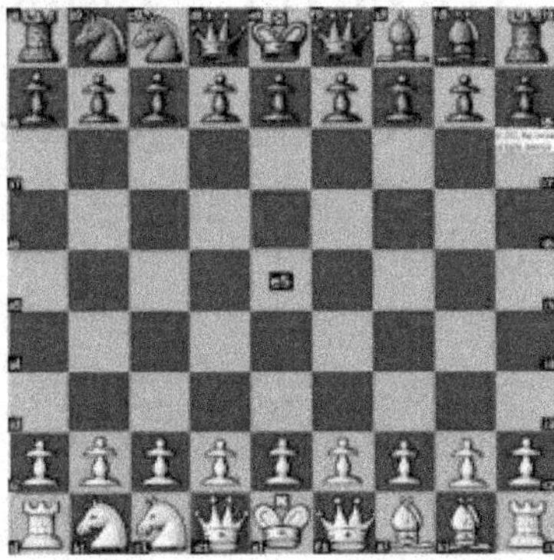

Play is identical to classical chess, with the following exceptions:

1. Each side has nine pawns instead of eight, and an extra queen.
2. The king can move two OR three squares when castling.
3. The fifty-move rule is extended to 1,000 moves.

These official rules must be updated in writing by Ray Gordon or his designated successor. Ray is the sole arbiter of all disputes in RG-99 until that time.

<u>Dated</u>: September 3, 2021

– Ray

Introduction:
The Ninth Key

Few, if any engines, would find the best, and perhaps the *only*, move in this position:

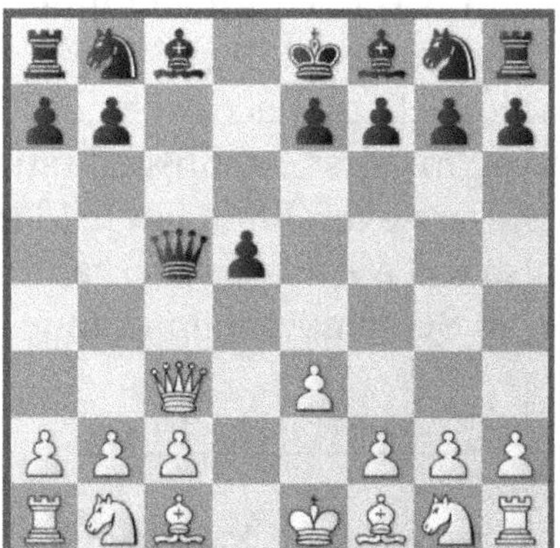

<u>*Moves*</u>: 1 e3 d5 2 d4 c5 3 cxd5 Qa5+ 4 Qd2! Qxc5 5 Qc3!

A similar position arises after 1 d4 d5 2 c4 dxc4 3 Qa4+ Qd7! 4 Qxa4 Qc6!, where the threat of 5 Qxc1+ forces the exchange of queens, just like the threat of 5…Qxc8+ does so here. No single position exemplifies the tunnel's radical shift from conventional opening theory, to what might – and ***should*** – become the dominant approach to chess openings: ***finding the lines which force a draw while maximizing reduction of the move tree through liquidation and transposition.*** This approach, placed on top of "normal" chess theory, gives total clarity to previously indecipherable opening positions, where central control, development, king safety and space take a backseat to the chess equivalent of a ***Pac-Man*** pattern: the drawing line, similar to what solved checkers.

<u>Pay Up</u>

My first established USCF rating was 1810, in September, 1987, was a good reflection of my ability, given my participation in the 1987 World Open (where former world champion GM Viswanathan Anand scored 6/9 as an IM at twenty!), and was also a clear signal to the chess world – particularly those who dished out Samford Fellowships – that I was also ***washed up***, simply ***too old*** to become world champion, for ***never a master at twenty-one*** was a unilateral disqualifier. In my case, however, my gaming youth was not wasted, for in addition to having won the Wagner Junior High School chess championship in 1981, without ever having cracked open a book, I had ***solved*** Pac-Man, in no small part because unlike chess, mistakes in video games cost $0.25 each, which adds up pretty quickly even for a working teenager who won a good deal of money at the track.

The resulting perfectionism of the financial pressure caused by having to cover retail space and electricity in the arcades made me a promising chessplayer in 1987, but, ironically, even much more so in 2023, when engines have all but turned chess into just another 1980s-style, ***solvable*** video game, a flaw so expensive to machine owners that future games were impossible to completely master. Only games like ***Qix, Paperboy,*** and my beloved ***Monaco GP*** had fixed time limits; regarding Qix, I'll have what the developers were having.

While chess offers no similar financial consequence for each mistake, my first teacher, Richard Gilmartin, used to threaten to terminate my "free" lessons if I didn't resign when lost, though this was a bit hollow as doing so would have cost him weed, pizza, and a seat at the table once the park filled up at Noon, on the few days he chose to remain after teaching me.   The lessons were an amazing bargain, and I was one of many future tournament players he helped morph from talented beginners into tournament killers. Unrated players in the park would use their estimated strength in their place: Richard placed me near 1800, but since it took six months of serious study in 1987 for 1810 to be my first established rating, I would estimate that in 1984 I was closer to 1700. I lost to rated players over 2000, but held my own against 1700 and under, so I was somewhere near there. I also did not have a tournament-strength opening repertoire, though I was definitely much closer in September than in June.

First Mistake Loses

"The contest is beginning to appear rigged." Larry Evans answered a reader's letter about how engine dominance in chess was a matter of hardware by that point (~1990) with a chilling warning to human players everywhere, on top of Deep Thought's rise to a 2525 rating by early 1989, a much more surprising quantum leap than subsequent advances that yielded Deep Blue, and today's engines like Stockfish and AlphaZero, now estimated to be well above 3500 in playing strength, about as close to perfection as one can achieve, or so we think.

As an "aspiring world champion" (basically adopting the persona of *The American* from the musical *Chess* to attract sapiosexual groupies, i.e., women turned on by intelligence), the future of chess, and the impact of engines on that future, preoccupied me: already "too old" to succeed, I was now faced with computers turning chess into *tic-tac-toe*, *Connect Four*, or what checkers would become: a forced draw (or win), with easily memorized, engine-created drawing lines ruining the game. It was also clear that there would be no comebacks, and that *perfect play from move <u>one</u>* was the only way a human could draw, though my Pac-Man experience suggested that while engines might one day become unbeatable, they'd never become <u>*undrawable*</u>: mistake-free human play could survive against anyone, even a pile of silicon.

Based on my experience with Pac-Man, including being the opponent in Bill Bastable's perfect game at an arcade at Sixty-First and First in July 1983, I fully expected humans to match engine play the same way we solved Pac-Man, but this was not to be: *forty* years later, and now more than a quarter century after Deep Blue defeated Kasparov, today's top players have simply thrown up their hands at the idea of drawing against engines, instead content to have *scripted exhibition matches* which are not technically rigged, but when you go fourteen moves in the main line of the Petroff (0.10), the likely outcome becomes overwhelmingly clear.

The tunnel is premised on chess being a forced draw, which means:

1. If all roads lead to 0.00, then *tree reduction* becomes the dominant evaluation factor, even if engines do not recognize it. For now, this creates a huge advantage, as engines miss moves like 3 Qd2/Qd7 above, as it "violates" conventional wisdom about development and early queen moves.

2. Beyond simplification and tree reduction, *liquidation* is next in importance, because in the course of learning how to weaponize the exchange of material, you'll master literally every chess skill needed to solve the game! Combined with making liquidation your primary option in any position, you'll wind up plugging up just about every weakness in your game, and your middlegame and endgame strength will go through the roof due to superior training positions.

Beyond these adjustments, chess theory remains completely intact, with the solution to checkers and its resulting drawing lines guiding the way. Complexity is fine if you wish to play intuitively, but a more methodical, efficient approach is far more likely to result in a higher rating. With that said, until we can completely memorize all drawing lines, at some point you'll have to play intuitively, relying on calculation and heuristics, the latter far more important as they will guide the former. It is these elements which separate the best players, who see things to which their mortal counterparts are completely blind, regardless of time control, and why *thinking hard* proves only that you don't know what you're doing: as Damon, a homeless man in Washington Square Park once told me, one day a player will make perfect moves without thinking; Damon was completely right, though his own play was about 1500 level on a good day.

Openings DO Matter!

Chess is 99.999% openings, and this has been proven throughout its history, with Bobby Fischer outbooking the world and gaining 900 points in two years (1726-2626 from 1955-1957), as he perfected a narrow repertoire. Kasparov used a quasi-tunnel involving the King's Indian formation and some selected systems involving 1. e4, including 9…Qa5+ against 9 Nd5 in the Pelikan Sicilian, forcing a draw in what used to be that main line, but from which White must deviate to avoid conceding the half-point that would cost him the world championship just as Kasparov was undone by the *Berlin Draw*, Kramnik's progenitor tunnel against the Ruy Lopez, but one which still left him vulnerable to the Center Game, Four Knights, Scotch, Bishop's Opening, Ponziani, and King's Gambit, among other deviations, all of which are sidestepped by the 1 e3/e6 tunnel.

Players who win with *trick openings* love to lecture about how openings don't matter, even as they collect most of their rating points from weak players who are fooled by the cheat:

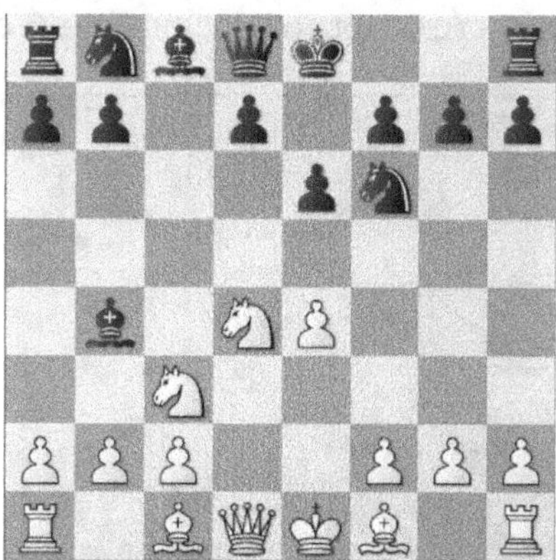

Moves: 1 e4 c5 2 Nf3 e6 3 d4 cxd4 4 Nxd4 Nf6 5 Nc3 Bb4

Legendary chess hustler Thomas D. "Tom" "Murph" Murphy (b. 1957) and I were two of maybe six people you could call at odd hours to find a high-level chessgame with an opponent rated 1800+. Even in New York, you'd have to find a place, as well as a player, but several all-night venues fit that bill for the most serious, who still formed a relatively small group. That I had air conditioning, food, and a place to crash made my apartment ideal not just for him, but for **Mate By Force**, the team of expert-rated Philadelphia hustlers assembled and personally trained by Emory Tate, father of Andrew Tate, a man with whom I shared a ride with on the way home in the 1987 World Open. Aside from the obligatory chest-thumping, we got along relatively well.

The Pin variation of the Sicilian is a typical hustler line, designed to exploit "book" play by White, at least in that era. The direct, primitive threat on e4 requires substantial positional knowledge to fend off, which most of Murph's marks, including me, were unable to do, until one night I gave a long look to the position, tired of playing 6. e5 (+0.78), as recommended by MCO and ECO, which I had just picked up. Modern engines endorse my "novelty," a move rarely played at the time, but one designed specifically to exploit Murph's materialism:

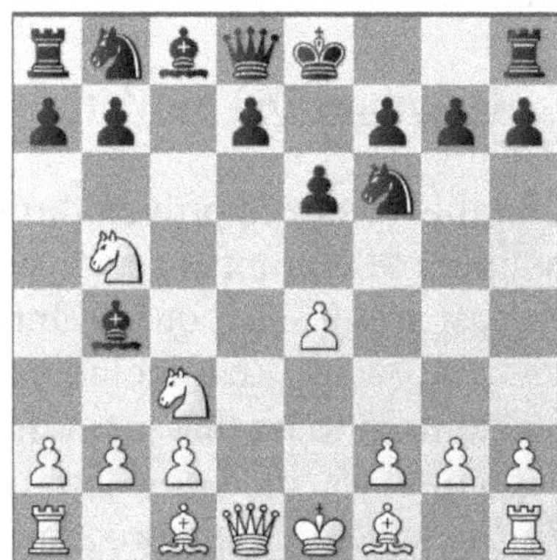

Moves: **1 e4 c5 2 Nf3 e6 3 d4 cxd4 4 Nxd4 Nf6 5 Nc3 Bb4 6 Ndb5!!**

The double-exclamation point is for shifting the battle from Murph's positional tricks to my tactical tricks, while demonstrating the clear material value of development. I *knew* how Murph would attack this line, and prepared a very special refutation, to score my first major win over my new sparring partner/coach. Murph grabbed the bait, as I knew he would, with 6…Nxe4 (1.44), now verified as a clear win for White, but other lines are still 0.20 or better, a perfect trap that does not compromise the position (except for eschewing 6 e5 for more familiar territory).

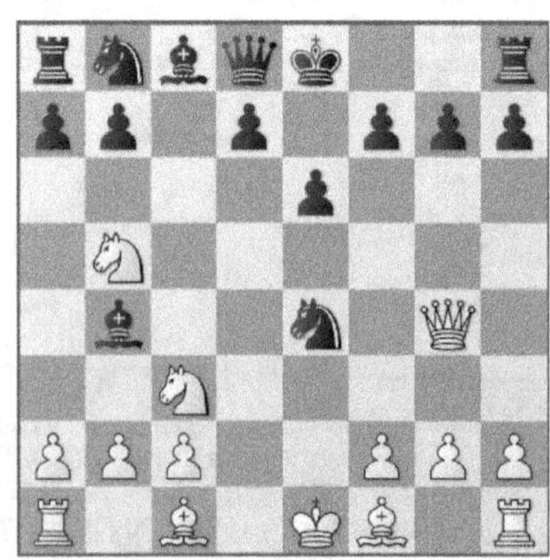

Moves: **1 e4 c5 2 Nf3 e6 3 d4 cxd4 4 Nxd4 Nf6 5 Nc3 Bb4 6 Ndb5 Nxe4 7 Qg4!!**

This ***motif*** occurs in numerous openings, and is critical knowledge for any tactician who enjoys a good sacrifice to achieve superior development, and which occurs frequently in the Winawer French, which I avoid like the plague, though I did toy around with 7. f4 in the main lines if only to see why it was rarely analyzed; I concluded it was sound. The silicon is damning against this ***trick opening:***

1. +/- (1.49): 7...Nxc3 8.bxc3 Bf8 9.Qg3 Na6 10.Bf4 b6 11.h4 Bb7 12.0-0-0 Rc8 13.Nd6+ Bxd6 14.Bxd6 Rg8 15.Bb5 Nc7 16.Bd3 g6 17.h5 Nd5 18.c4 Nf6 19.hxg6 hxg6 20.Rh3 Rc6 21.f3 Nh5 22.Qh2 Rxd6 23.Qxd6 Qg5+ 24.Kb1 Qf4 25.Qa3 a5 26.Be4 Bxe4 27.fxe4 Qc7 28.Qc3 Ke7 29.Qd2 Nf4 30.Rb3 e5 31.Qf2 Ne6 32.Qxb6

2. +- (2.02): 7...d5 8.Qxg7 Rf8 9.Bf4 Na6 10.a3 Bxc3+ 11.bxc3 Qf6 12.Qxf6 Nxf6 13.Rb1 Kd7 14.Be2 Ne8 15.c4 Nac7 16.Nxc7 Nxc7 17.Rd1 b6 18.cxd5 exd5 19.0-0 Re8 20.Bd3 Kc6 21.Rfe1 h5 22.Rxe8 Nxe8 23.c4 Nc7 24.cxd5+ Nxd5

3. +- (2.45): 7...Nc6 8.Qxg7 Ke7 9.a3 Rg8 10.Qh6 Bxc3+ 11.Nxc3 Nxc3 12.Bg5+ Rxg5 13.Qxg5+ Ke8 14.Qxd8+ Kxd8 15.bxc3 b6 16.0-0-0 Ke7 17.g4 Ne5 18.Rg1 Ng6 19.Rd4 e5 20.Bg2 Rb8 21.Re1 d6 22.Rc4 Kf6 23.Bf3 Bb7 24.Be2 Nf4 25.Rc7 h6 26.Bc4 d5 27.Bb3 Ne6 28.Rd7 Nf8 29.Rd6+ Ne6 30.Bxd5 Ke7 31.Rxe6+ fxe6 32.Bxb7 Rxb7 33.Rxe5 Rc7 34.Kb2 Rc4 35.h3

4. +- (2.48): 7...0-0 8.Qxe4 Nc6 9.Nd4 Rb8 10.Nxc6 bxc6 11.Qe5 d6 12.Qg3 f5 13.Bc4 Kh8 14.a3 Ba5 15.0-0 e5 16.f4 Bb6+ 17.Kh1 d5 18.Be2 d4 19.Na4 e4 20.b4 Qf6 21.Qg5 Qd6 22.Rd1 Bd8 23.Qg3 Bf6 24.Bb2 Rd8 25.Bxd4 Bxd4 26.c3 c5 27.Nxc5 Bxc5 28.Rxd6 Bxd6 29.Qg5 Be6

5. +- (2.63): 7...f5 8.Qxg7 Rf8 9.Be2 Qf6 10.Qxf6 Rxf6 11.0-0 Na6 12.Nxe4 fxe4 13.c4 d5 14.a3 Be7 15.Be3 dxc4 16.Bxc4 Bd7 17.Rac1 Rf5 18.Nd4 Rf6 19.Be2 Rc8 20.Rxc8+ Bxc8 21.Nb5 Bd7 22.b4 Rf5 23.Nc3 Nc7 24.Bg4 Rf8 25.Rd1 b6 26.h3 Nd5 27.Nxd5 exd5 28.Bxd7+ Kxd7 29.Rxd5+ Bd6 30.Rh5 Rf7 31.g3

6. +- (2.96): 7...a6 8.Qxe4 Be7 9.Nd4 d5 10.Qe3 Bf6 11.Be2 Nc6 12.Nxc6 bxc6 13.Qd2 e5 14.0-0 0-0 15.b3 Rb8 16.Na4 Re8 17.Qd1 Qd6 18.c3 e4 19.Be3 Be5 20.g3 Bh3 21.Re1 Qg6 22.Bh5 Qf5 23.Rc1 Re6 24.f4

7. +- (3.14): 7...Ba5 8.Qxe4 d5 9.Qg4 0-0 10.Qg3 Kh8 11.Bf4 Nc6 12.0-0-0 a6 13.Nd4 f6 14.Bd6 Re8 15.Nb3 Bxc3 16.bxc3 Bd7 17.f4 a5 18.Ba3 Ne7 19.Nd4 b5 20.Bxb5 Bxb5 21.Nxb5 Qb6 22.Nd6 Reb8 23.c4 Nf5 24.Nxf5

The ridiculous level of today's engine analysis was unavailable in 1987, so I had to figure out for myself if the line was sound, as well as how to punish Murph's overextensive pawn grab. I knew one mistake would result in defeat and a condescending lecture about how booking up is bad. ***"You play the first twelve moves like a champ and fall apart,"*** was Murph's correct assessment of my play, but we diverged when I noted that it was much easier to learn how to close out winning positions than it was to get them, and that eventually my technique would catch up, and my rating would surpass his. Thirty-six years later, we are still having this debate, with no clear winner, as our ratings are still relatively similar, no small feat at our ages.

Murph didn't even play these lines, instead falling into more of my anticipated traps with 7...Bxc3? 8 bxc3 Nf6 9 Qxg7 Rg8:

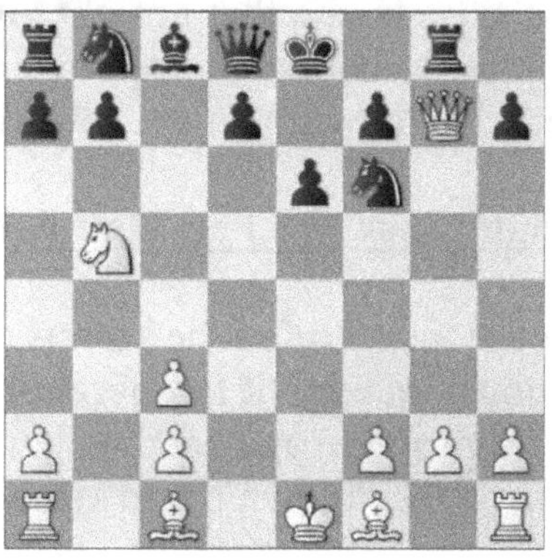

Ray-Murph After 9…Rg8??

After 10 Nd6+!!, Black is sunk. Murph went ahead and helpmated himself via *double check* (one of many motifs I learned in Washington Square Park from Richard Gilmartin) with 10…Ke7 11 Ba3!! Rxg7 12 Nf5+ Ke8 13 Nxe7#, a *signature game* which established our lifelong chess rivalry. The game also defined what would become my signature style of the pre-engine era, where developmental sacrifices occurred frequently. Almost every move exemplifies the power of ignoring overextension in the opening, and letting the opponent waste time (moves) on captures while deploying the army at warp speed for a quick, crushing win. As a general rule, three developmental tempi equals one pawn, but the engines have found many notable exceptions.

Today, I would not allow the Pin Variation because 1 e4 requires too much engine preparation, as just the Sicilian has many alternatives for Black instead of the standard Open Sicilian, itself containing several main lines, all of which White must master, against an opponent with a designer engine line just off the beaten path, which s/he will know much better than you, turning the entire game, and a large part of your rating, into a test of some obscure line rather than actual chess theory and its execution. By focusing on tree reduction and liquidation literally from move one, the tunnel is all but impossible to avoid or take out of book, assuring invincibility in the opening, freeing my time to focus on middlegames, endgames, and tactics.

While I loved being able to take the fight to Murph from move one, leading to games which drew large crowds in *LOVE Park* (back when we had to hunt down an opponent), the scripted openings which Fischer claimed were the death of chess still have a large place in modern chess theory, but much more selectively, and only in lines which can result from 1 e3/e6, the open Sicilian seemingly not one of them, but other tunnels could be created which transpose into them. I still play several main line openings, but only after sidestepping the tricks and traps in every line via my highly flexible and restrictive first move, one first revealed to me as likely best after the research which led to *960 Stems*, still the only single-volume reference for Chess960.

Just to be clear, I can still play intuitively, but this is rating suicide today, as it requires several times more preparation and study that some players might be able to pull off, but even they would do better with the tunnel. Even my previous attempts at tree reduction were too easy to target: the Ponziani still left me open to the Elephant, Petroff, Philidor, and Latvian, as well as all the other replies to 1 e4, all of which I could avoid with 1 e3, a move which also achieved symmetry with 1 e6, allowing for even more *tree reduction*, by playing identical openings with colors reversed, with or without the extra tempo that I might give back: e.g., 1 e3 b6 2 e4!!, to get the same position as 1 b3 e5, a priority not recognized by engines, yet clearly best for any player seeking familiarity and tree reduction with an eye towards a forced draw.

<u>Drawing Lines Are Pac-Man Patterns</u>

Mastering Pac-Man, by Ken Uston, revealed the secrets of the *Ninth Key*, the board where the game's titular character slows down, making it far more difficult to derive a monster-evading pattern that leads to a forced draw (high score) against the engine (game). Bill Bastable took this to another level, claiming three dots on the "blown board" (the 256th), where the game resets, and one Pac-Man is sacrificed to claim each dot, for a perfect score. Uston effectively ended the Pac-Man craze, supplanted by the supposedly unsolvable ***Ms. Pac Man,*** with "random" monster patterns that Bastable tore apart in no time flat, leading developers to abandon solvable games in favor of combat scenarios or fixed-time games like ***Monaco GP***, while video-enhanced pinball (with ***multi-ball!***) injected new life into my old arcade favorite.

When I finally migrated to chess in late 1986, mostly due to Kate's gift of the score from ***Chess*** almost two years earlier, the rise of chess engines was well underway, leading me to purchase the ***Fidelity 2100,*** a brilliant tactician, but no threat to the elite. Having already been given ***Chess Challenger*** and the surprisingly strong Atari chess cartridge, I was familiar with engine-aided play, particularly in solving complex tactical openings like the Poisoned Pawn Sicilian and Four Pawns Alekhine, and my beloved Muzio Gambit, the first opening I ever studied in Washington Square Park, but tree reduction made these lines unplayable, something I had not foreseen when I first conceived the tunnel in 1989 as an antidote for perfect engine play.

Engines have reduced chess to memorization, with the tunnel aiming for maximum simplification via tree reduction, liquidation, and transposition whenever possible. These priorities allow me to uncover moves which are clearly best, yet buried among several seemingly equivalent alternatives, all of which require ten times the prep. Not playing 3...Qd7 in the QGA as shown earlier is tantamount to assigning yourself four times the homework to achieve the same 0.00 to which all roads lead. Since engines are now strong enough for their evaluations to be determinative, the drawing lines I envisioned in 1989 have begun taking shape, though a portion of the late-stage jigsaw puzzle, that gets easier the more it is pieced together, remains to be solved.

High-Intensity Bodybuilding

In late 1993, a woman rejected me because I was overweight, among other reasons. As this was easiest to fix, I resolved to be in perfect shape come springtime, and to zip past her on my skates, which I did, my weight down from 225 to 183 pounds, and my bodyfat to an all-time low of 11.7 percent. It would take five years for my weight to recross 210 pounds, and another two to reach 230, where I stayed at for a while before completely letting go, only to lose back the weight with age and some health concerns. The looks novelty wore off, and I was attracting more women than I knew what to do with, so my incentive was gone. What remains, however, is the lesson from Ellington Darden's book of the same name as the header, a training method which allowed me to make more progress in four months than I had in several years prior.

Darden's masterpiece taught me to question conventional wisdom, and to find logical solutions on my own, as I had set out to do with my ambitious fitness goals of the ***Winter of Twenty-Seven***, defined by its seventeen ice storms which had me in hibernation when not taking advantage of thermoregulation in cold weather to accelerate my weight loss, my goal of 183 pounds having been achieved in mid-March. The high-intensity program was just that: three (later two) intense, full-body workouts each week, rather than alternating half the body every day, allowing for bigger rips that fill during the convalescence between workouts. My results were similar to what I'm now experiencing with the tunnel: this is simply ***the correct way to train, at least for me***. If you are stuck with developing your own method, try this one first.

One:
The Fine Art Of Transposition (Key Positions)

While many transpositions occur naturally and are discovered accidentally, true weaponization of this art form will serve you well. Here's a position from 1989:

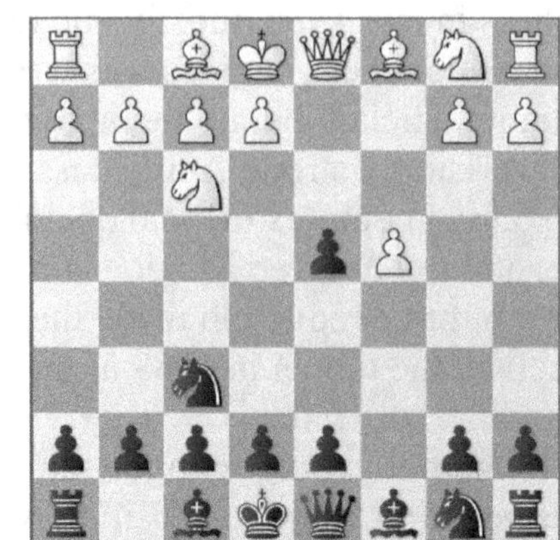

Moves: **1 d4 Nf6 2 c4 c5 3 Nf3 exd4**
1 c4 Nf6 2 d4 c5 3 Nf3 exd4
1 Nf3 c5 2 d4 Nf6 3 c4 exd4
1 Nf3 Nf6 2 c4 c5 3 d4 exd4
1 Nf3 c5 2 c4 Nf6 3 d4 exd4
1 Nf3 Nf6 2 d4 c5 3 c4 exd4

Six different move orders lead to a *key position*, from which variations and transpositions are then used to reach *key #2*, #3 and beyond, until the drawing line is completely fleshed out. As I like to say, *I don't pick my moves; they pick me*, and they do. The additional priorities of tree reduction, liquidation, and transposition rarely leave more than one or two moves as clearly best, whereas engines might give you ten or more seemingly equal alternatives; this is where allegedly strong players go to lose.

The QGA Key

A good key will have several entrance lanes, where the game "begins" several moves in:

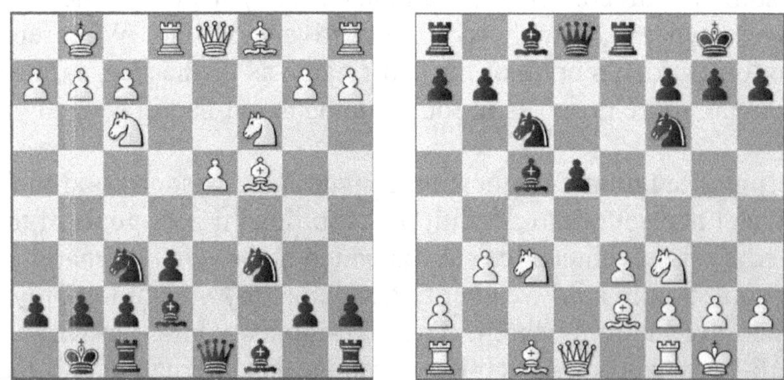

Black QGA Key After 9…Nc6   **White QGA Key after 10 b3!**

Moves: 1 d4 e6 2 c4 d5 3 Nf3 dxc4 4 e3 c5 5 Bxc4 cxd4 6 exd4 Nf6 7 O-O Be7 8 Nc3 O-O 9 Re1 Nc6 (b)
1 e3 d5 2 d4 c5 3 dxc5 e6 4 c4 Bxc5 5 cxd5 exd5 6 Nf3 Nf6 7 Nc3 O-O 8 Be2 Nd6 9 O-O Re8 10 b3! (w)

The ***key components*** are moves which are almost entirely interchangeable; the exclamation point is for familiarity after 10 b3, or 10…b6 in almost every line for Black, combining for an awesome weapon for either side, with incredible familiarity and tree reduction in one of the game's most complex openings. Expect a brutal learning curve: I got slaughtered for one year with this opening, and took another two before I arrived at the ***solution*** you see here, after which the engines take over and will expand your perfect play all the way to the forced draw if you stay the course, especially if you are much younger than me. You will also pick up many wins along the way, as I did in fifteen moves with Black against GM Anton Korobov (2688), at the time ranked #42 in the world, which almost prompted my retirement, as I might never top this.

The Rubinstein French Key

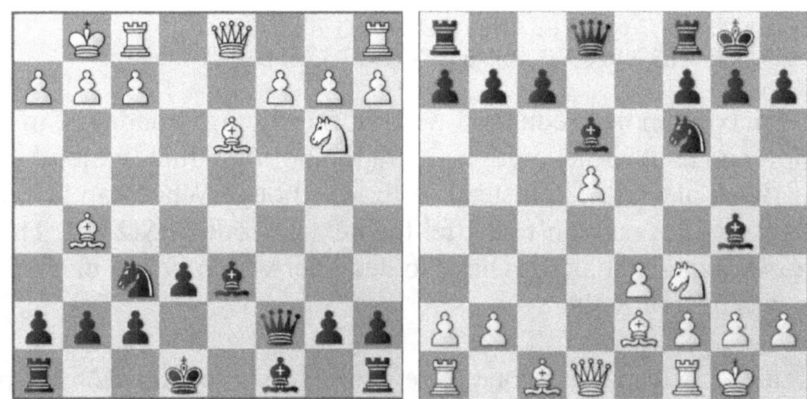

Rubinstein Key After 12…Qc7 (b)   Rubinstein Key After 10 cxd5 (w)

Moves: 1 e4 e6 2 d4 d5 3 Nc3 dxe4 4 Nxe4 Nd7 5 Nf3 Ngf6 6 Bxf6 Nf6 7 Bd3 c5 8 O-O cxd4 9 Nxd4 Bc5 10 Nb3 Bd6 11 Bg5 Qc7 (b)
 1 e3 e5 2 d4 Nc6 3 dxe5 Nxe5 4 Nd2 Nf6 5 Ngf3 Nxf3+ 6 Nxf3 d5 7 Be2 Bd6 8 O-O O-O 9 c4 Bg4 10 cxd5 (w)

For Black, the key occurs frequently, with most deviations leading to positions governed by similar heuristics and motifs, while White has the luxury of cutting off the key, since 10…Nxd5 runs into 11 Qxd5!! Bxh2+ 12 Nxh2 Qxd5 13 Nxg4 (0.45), leading to a still-playable, but highly imbalanced position for Black, and a game that, once the key is mastered, ***begins at move twelve,*** at which point the engines should make forcing the draw a relatively simple matter of technique for an elite player. Other main lines, like the Petroff, have keys this far into the game, but the same cannot be said for the King's Gambit, Bishop's Opening, Center Game, and any other obscure second move for White. The tunnel is immune to this type of manipulation.

Unlike most opening repertoires, the tunnel will lead you straight to the main line of one of several different openings, with far fewer, much weaker, and less complicated detours, with overlapping motifs, and its use of 1 e3 allows for extra transposition between Black and White, either with the extra tempo, to achieve even greater tree reduction by cutting off the most complicated lines.

The Exchange French Key

By far, the most frequently occurring line is the Exchange French, which I can play from either side, with or without the extra tempo as White. Those who think this hair-splitting variation is a drawish line have never played it; it is definitely drawish, but only when mastered:

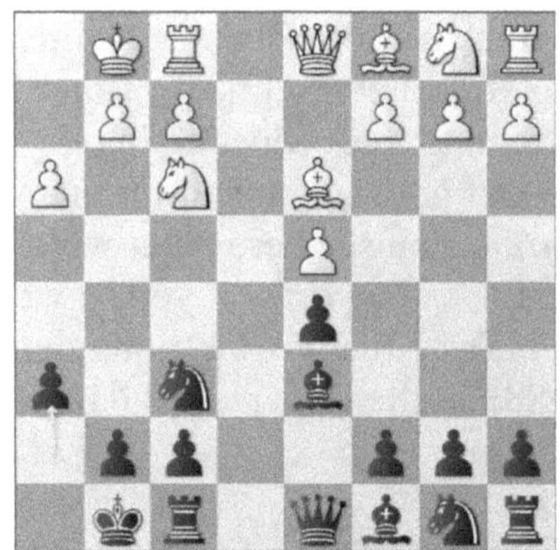
Exchange French Key After 7…h6 (b/w)

**Moves**: 1 e4 e6 2 d4 d5 3 exd5 exd5 4 Nf3 Nf6 5 Bd3 Bd6 6 O-O O-O 7 h3 h6 (b)
      1 e4 e6 2 d4 d5 3 exd5 exd5 4 h3 Nf6 5 Nf3 Bd6 6 Bd3 O-O 7 O-O h6 (w)

Once again, we get maximum tree reduction without sacrificing soundness, in a key that can be reached from either color, and another key with an extra tempo for White (which I use to play 4. h3 to cut off the Bg4 lines) if Black plays 1…e6 instead of 1…e5, though White can give Black "White" with 2 e4! against 1…e6. Confused? You won't be after the next episode of **_SOAP!_** This line is a lot like the scene in **_Tango & Cash,_** where the heroes have to decipher which image in a hall-of-mirrors symmetrical nightmare was the real villain.

From here, the engines can lead you to one of several options for **_Key #2._** My personal preferences are in my free downloadable repertoire (linked here and the current version through my internet channels), and currently run towards Nc6-Ne7, with the idea of c6 and Bf5, or the equivalent moves for White. Consequently, I am stopping the key analysis here, though this line is such that, once mastered, you'll find yourself on auto-pilot all the way to the early endgame, at which point the real fun begins, with excellent drawing chances against any level of player, or even the strongest engines, none of which can impose a defeat against perfect play.

The Advance French Key

This line, like its inventor (Aron Nimzowitsch), is deceptively annoying, and has a very short key:

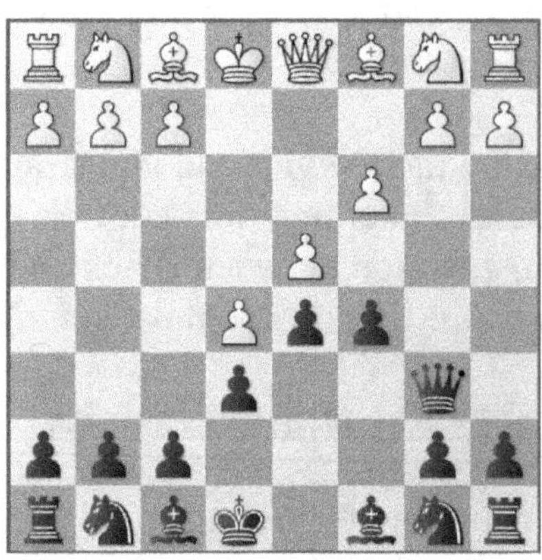
Advance French Key After 5 c3

The Slav/Caro Key

All tunnel lines have humble beginnings, and while I can and do win with intuitive play in this line, White is playing for a very small, very solid, persistent advantage that is no threat to the elite player, and is also a good measuring stick for your technique, since that is what will almost always win the day. Many grandmasters have taken to aiming for Bd7-Bb5 and liquidation of the "bad" (actually just defensive) Bishop, but Black usually has stronger, and must also learn to deal with a few highly complex but unfavorable detours along the way, mostly involving 4 Qg4. Despite the short nature of this key, Black has achieved a lot and defined the battle on his terms, huge steps towards forcing a draw with Black, all but assuring victory in a world title match.

The QGA and French keys cover most major lines for Black (and White), and even overlap themselves when dxc4/dxc5 is played, with the advantage of the undeveloped c-pawn. Another key with many similar motifs is the exchange Slav/Caro:

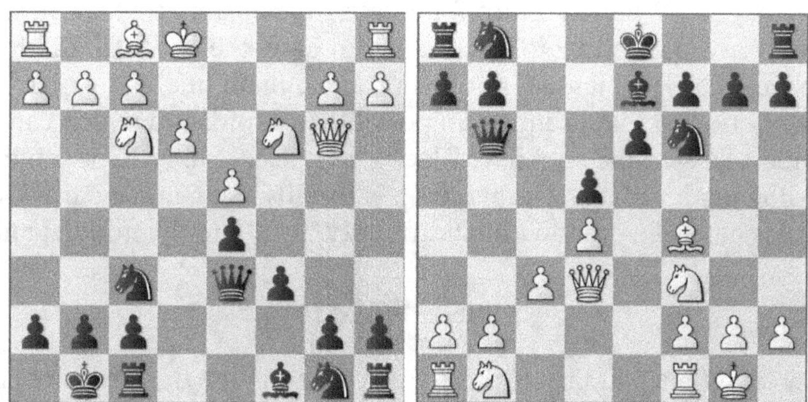

Slav Tunnel After 9 Qb3 (b)   Slav Tunnel After 9…Be7 (w)

**Moves**: 1 d4 e6 2 c4 d5 3 cxd5 exd5 4 Nc3 c6 5 Bf4 Bd6 6 Bxd6 Qxd6 7 Nf3 Nf6 8 e3 O-O 9 Qb3 Bf5 (b)
      1 e3 c5 2 d4 cxd4 3 exd4 d5 4 c3 Nf6 5 Bf4 Bf5 6 Bd3 Bxd3 7 Qxd3 Qb6 8 Nf3 e6 9 O-O Be7 (w)

These tunnels are slightly different, since White's extra tempo allows for the **_poisoned pawn_** sacrifice Qxb2, while giving White a leg up in castling. Don't be fooled, however: technique is paramount here, given the highly fluid, ambiguous nature of the position. You may have difficulty with this line long after others become your **_rating ATM_**, but this is nothing to fear, and another good test of your intuition, technique, and mastery of heuristics and motifs, of which there are many here. Though **_creativity_** is a cuss word these days, as it implies lack of memorization of the silicon oracle's wisdom, openings like this are fast becoming its last bastion, a harkening to the days when players could construct plans on the fly.

The Meran Key

The catch-all approach to hypermodern lines picked me; I certainly never would have chosen this line, as I never even knew what the Meran system was, let alone studied it enough to weaponize it for tournament play, but the tunnel has forced me to become rather well-versed in what turns out to be one of the most straightforward openings in the game, another one which can be played from either side:

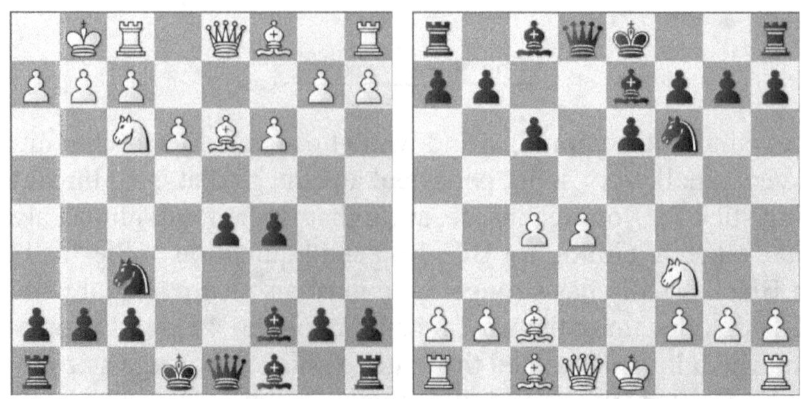

Meran Key After 10…Bc7 (b)   **Meran Key After 10 Bc2 (w)**

<u>*Moves*</u>: 1 d4 e6 2 e3 d5 3 c3 Nf6 4 Nf3 c5 5 Bd3 Nc6 6 O-O Bd6 7 Nbd2 e5 8 dxe5 Nxe5 9 Nxe5 Bxe5 10 Nf3 Bc7 (b)
1 e3 d5 2 d4 e6 3 c4 c6 4 Nf3 Nf6 5 Nc3 Be7 6 Bd3 Nbd7 7 e4 dxe4 8 Nxe4 Nxe4 9 Bxe4 Nf6 10 Bc2 (w)

This line is critical for tunnelers because it is almost a default for passive players as Black, conceding a slight advantage to White in return for a defensive posture that is extremely difficult to crack. White deliberately avoids castling to set a trap with h4 in the event Black strays from the forced draw, allowing a decisive Bxh7+, which does not work in the main line, but which does accomplish massive tree reduction after a key that is almost impossible to avoid, and which can be played nearly identically from any side. To stop the sacrifice, Black needs access to Nf6, or some other means of blunting the attack. Allowing e5/e4 against this setup is usually fatal, and even if the correct line is played, the tunneler holds at least a draw without difficulty, well into the middlegame.

Fianchetto Keys

While there are several fianchetto keys, most are covered in the third-rank openings below. The most frequently occurring key is also the most thematic: the KID key.

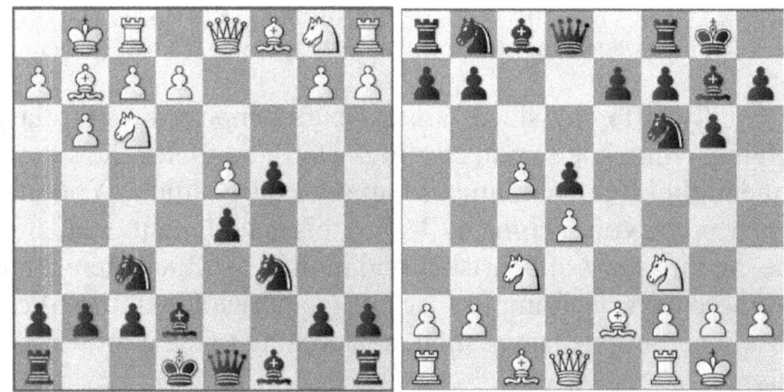

KID Key After 8…c4 (b)   **KID Key After 9 c5 (w)**

<u>*Moves*</u>: 1 g3 e6 2 Bg2 d5 3 Nf3 c5 4 O-O Nf6 5 d3 Nc6 6 c4 Be7 7 cxd5 exd5 8 d4 c4 (b)
1 e3 g6 2 d4 Bg7 3 Nf3 Nf6 4 c4 O-O 5 Be2 d6 6 Nc3 c5 7 O-O cxd4 8 exd4 d5 9 c5 (w)

The keys are not entirely similar, but they are also superfluous, since 1 g3 e5! and 1 e3 g6 2 e4! avoid these lines, at the cost of giving "White" to Black in exchange for remaining deep within engine preparation for a huge edge in familiarity. This is an alternative path, or spur.

Third-Rank Keys

Each key will be analyzed in depth in its own chapter. With these keys, White has given up the extra tempo to reach an ***identical*** position with either color, within the tunnel:

- **Larsen:**   1 b3 e5 (b)
                       1 e3 b6 2 e4! (w)

- **Hypermodern:**   1 g3 e5 (b)
                       1 e3 g6 2 e4! (w)

- **Pirc/KID:**   1 d3 e5 (b)
                       1 e3 d6 2 e4! (w)

Big Center Keys

When your opponent does not contest the center, the three-pawn or even four-pawn center is on the table, and is worth grabbing so frequently that I begin singing ***Push It!*** to remind myself of this, while giving one last look to the alternatives:

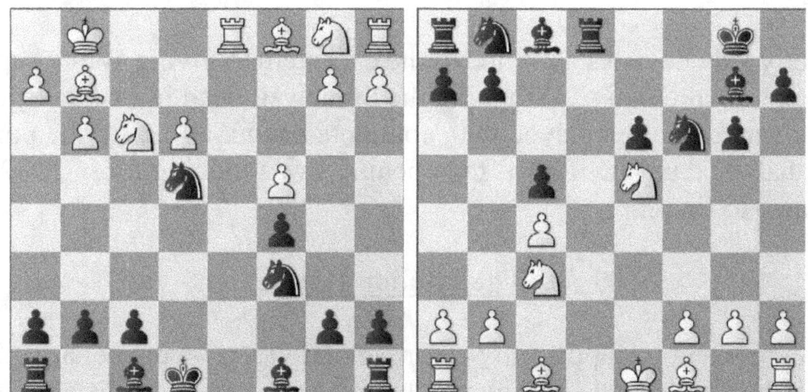

Big Center Key After 10…Nxe4 (b)   **Big Center Key After 11 Nxe5 (w)**

Moves: 1 d3 e5 2 g3 d5 3 Bg2 c5 4 c4 d4 5 Nf3 Nc6 6 O-O Nf6 7 e3 dxe3 8 fxe3 e4 9 dxe4 Qxd1 10 Rxd1 Nxe4 (b)
         1 e3 d6 2 e4 g6 3 d4 Bg7 4 c4 c5 5 d5 Nf6 6 Nc3 O-O 7 Nf3 e6 8 dxe6 fxe6 9 e5 dxe5 10 Qxd8 Rxd8 11 Nxe5 (w)

The big-center keys are excellent drawing lines once you've mastered techniques for continuing closed systems. Maneuvering underneath the space advantage to rearrange your army into an ideal formation, opening one or more lines for your well-placed pieces, and ***patience*** are keys to winning, with at least the draw in hand. Such passive play is nothing to fear, and a properly prepared initiative will make you very difficult to stop as the game wears on. Once again, using the same systems with White or Black greatly reduces the move tree, while doubling the mileage and frequency of the engine prep.

The Horsefly Key

I lost the final round of the under-1400 section of the 1987 World Open because I played 1…d5 against the Bird, allowing my opponent a Stonewall setup. For years, I remained convinced that my decision not to play the From Gambit was fatal, but instead it was my ignorance of the amazing power of the Horsefly defense:

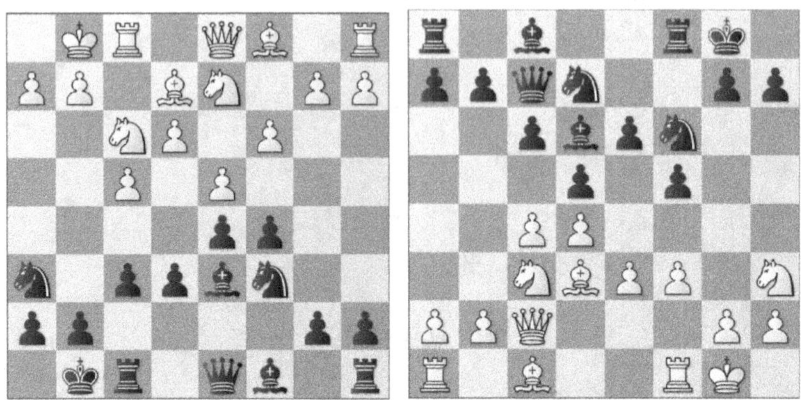

Horsefly Key After 8…f6 (b)   **Horsefly Key After 9…Qc7 (w)**

*Moves***:** 1 f4 Nh6 2 e3 e6 3 d4 d5 4 c3 c5 5 Nd2 Nc6 6 Ngf3 Bd6 7 Be2 O-O 8 O-O f6 (b)
  1 e3 f5 2 Nh3 e6 3 d4 d5 4 c4 c6 5 Nc3 Nf6 6 Qc2 Bd6 7 Bd3 O-O 8 O-O Nbd7 9 f3 Qc7 (w)

The White Horsefly Key deviates a bit due to the extra tempo giving White superior options to mirroring, which remains an alternative. Stopping the Stonewall dead in its tracks jams up the opponent's tunnel-like opening, often played with complete *tunnel vision*, to the point of implosion when forced into the analytical abyss. *This* is the opening I was looking for in 1987, and it took only three decades and change to find it!

The London Key

Setting aside for a moment my apparently controversial views on the negative impact on the gene pool of those who play the intellectual abomination known as the London system, I use two tunnels, the first a bit radical, and the second a relatively easy draw once mastered (no small feat). After 1 d4 e6 2 Bf4 *g5!?* (0.63), Black has flipped the familiarity script while still holding a tenuous draw, and the White version 1 e3 d5 2 d4 Bf5 3 g4 (-0.11), achieves practical equality in a line London players generally try to avoid, but cannot. The more traditional tunnel arises in other lines as well:

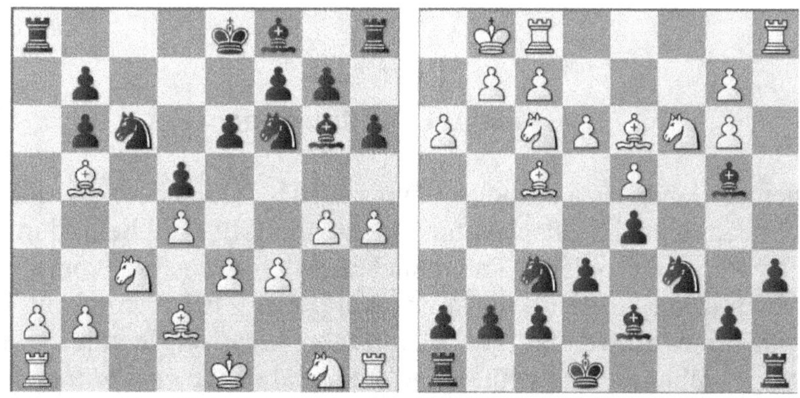

London Key After 12 Bd2 (w)   **London Key After 12 O-O (b)**

<u>*Moves:*</u> 1 e3 d5 2 d4 c6 3 c4 Bf5 4 Qb3 Qb6 5 Qxb6 axb6 6 cxd5 cxd5 7 Nc3 e6 8 Bb5+ Nc6 9 f3 Nf6 10 g4 Bg6 11 h4 h6 12 Bd2 (w)
1 d4 e6 2 Bf4 d5 3 Nf3 c5 4 c3 Qb6 5 Qb3 cxd4 6 cxd4 Qxb3 7 axb3 Nc6 8 Nc3 Nf6 9 e3 Bb4 10 Bd3 Bd7 11 h3 a6 12 O-O (b)

The moves are similar, and mostly interchangeable, leading to dead equality from a position the engines can carry into tablebase territory, if not to the end of the forced-drawing line. Over time, you'll work out your own key (or use this one), with similar motifs and engine evaluations, in positions where the Queens are rapidly liquidated, making a win almost impossible to achieve against proper technique with tunnel-level familiarity, the latter only coming with time, as in *years* of practice and rehearsal, though rating improvement will occur much sooner. What you won't do is *stop* improving your rating because today's losses and draws will turn into tomorrow's draws and wins, as the remaining pieces of the jigsaw puzzle grow fewer.

Other openings, even the Sokolski and Grob, lend themselves more to intuitive play, while the former drops a pawn when played in reverse. The Grob is a forced win for Black, which any elite player should have no difficulty destroying on instinct and heuristics, even though many do. The heart and soul of the tunnel, however, are the dozen or so keys outlined above, all of which cut homework in half while doubling the mileage thanks to their being played by either color, making invincibility in the opening relatively simple to achieve, greatly increasing familiarity with the middlegame and endgame, and which for me has yielded my best *return on training* ever. Constructing tunnels to keys for these openings can be done, but is not necessary, and won't impact your rating much. Even if you wind up playing against these openings to the point of impacting your rating, a simple stem can be constructed in a few hours or less.

Impressive as the above may seem, it only scratches the surface of what is possible with transposition, and with each key having several entrance ramps, your rating will improve sharply as you weaponize transposition rather than just marveling at how to turn an Exchange French into a favorable QGA, a Caro-Kan into a Classical French, or even a From Gambit into a King's Gambit. Key positions were noted by me as a means of circumventing the need to memorize specific lines, when almost all roads to that position are paved with the same moves in varying order. From my humble observation that the Rubinstein French took out the Tarrasch while simultaneously neutralizing the Classical and liquidating the center, to my failed experiment with a d3/d6 tunnel a few years ago, my decision to bite the bullet and master the e3/e6 tunnel has paid off huge, and will continue to do so for the relatively brief remainder of my career, and, for younger readers so choose, the extremely long remainder of yours.

Two:
The Fine Art Of Liquidation

The Blackmar-Diemer Gambit is a dubious pawn sacrifice which barely holds the draw for White, while presenting numerous practical headaches for Black, who falls well behind in development, but who can also neutralize without a problem. The tunnel allows for mostly favorable transpositions against this opening, which is very difficult for any player under 2400 to confront, but which is not a concern as one's technique rises above that level. Until then, however, lectures about openings not mattering when in fact it is technique that is the issue is typical of the ***gaslighting*** faced by rapidly improving players whose repertoire is much stronger than their technique, a temporary condition which will rectify itself over time. Here, however, a quote about the Gambit from GM Joe Gallagher is relevant to liquidation:

> *"[O]nce there is no attack and the position looks rather balanced they tend to assess the game as equal, <u>forgetting the fact that they are a pawn down.</u>"*

Winning this pawn-up position is a critical skill for the tunneler, or any player who wishes not to convert forced wins into draws or losses. The first position presented here was a line from the QGA where liquidation of queens is forced on move ***three***. Anytime Black (or even White) can simplify the position towards an endgame with draw in hand (a common tactic of former world champion Magnus Carlsen), they have achieved the goal of the tunnel, and reduced the game to an endgame battle in which they are substantially more familiar with the terrain.

Liquidating a winning position a clear pawn up is a matter of technique that will develop naturally, but the process of liquidating itself is what will help your game the most, since this will require knowledge of literally every corner of chess theory. Much more important are the exchanges which occur with even material, which simplify into winning positions, or which convert to positional advantages.

<u>Chess Losing Against Checkers</u>

The impossibility of playing chess against checkers aside, people love to treat the former as "stronger," yet there are notable exceptions.

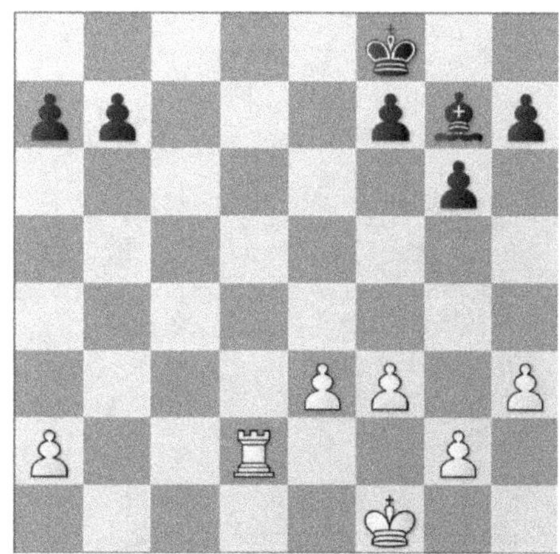

White To Play And Win

White creates a ***checkerboard*** with 1. e4 and 2. Rd5, after which Black's king is boxed in, and his bishop permanently muted, allowing the White king free run of the board, to mop up Black's queenside pawns, and win easily. Liquidation into a favorable king-and-pawn ending also looms large once White has ideally positioned his king:

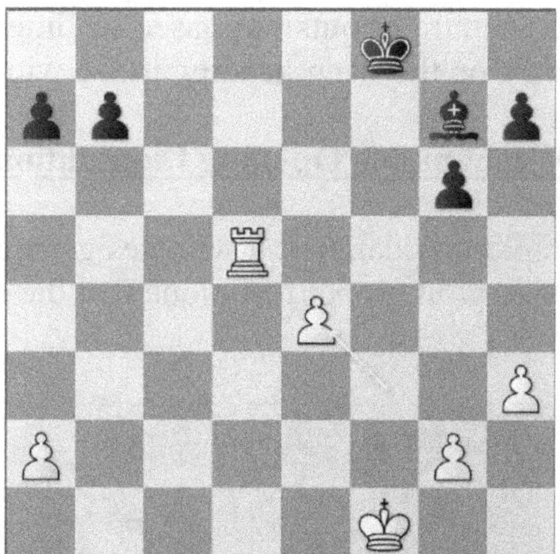

Easy Win After 1 e4 f5 2 Rd5 fxe4 3 fxe4

White becomes completely unstoppable here, in a setup which is relatively easy to establish, particularly by the player aware of its strength who points towards it from earlier rather than just stumbling upon it. This is one of many ***endgame tunnels*** you can use to return to forcing territory, in this case to simplify a win.

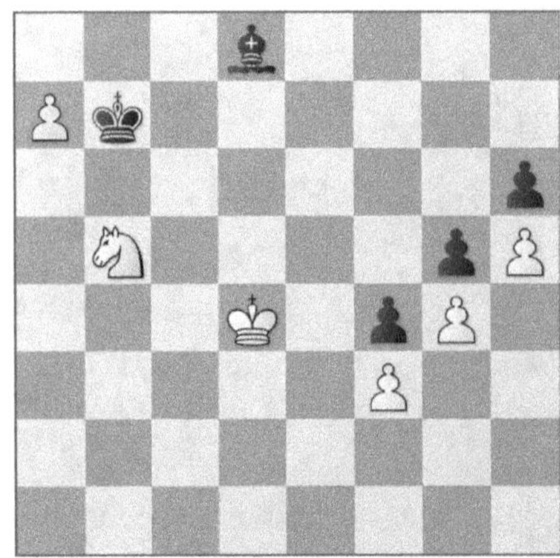

White Wins

More convoluted versions of this motif can be found in Kasparyan's ***Domination in 2,545 Endgame Studies***, perhaps the best chess book ever written, and certainly the best endgame book, replete with mostly contrived positions which still confound the engines.

Liquidation should always be favorable, either by locking up the board when up a rook against a bishop, or by tying a major piece to an extra or outside passer, leading to liquidation that leaves your king in the center and your opponent's on the wing, leading to the win of multiple pawns.

<u>**Weaponizing Opening Liquidation**</u>

Some openings are based on rapid liquidation that violates general principles, but which leads to positions where the draw is easily held with proper technique that the opponent often lacks, particularly in the Black Lion or its relatives:

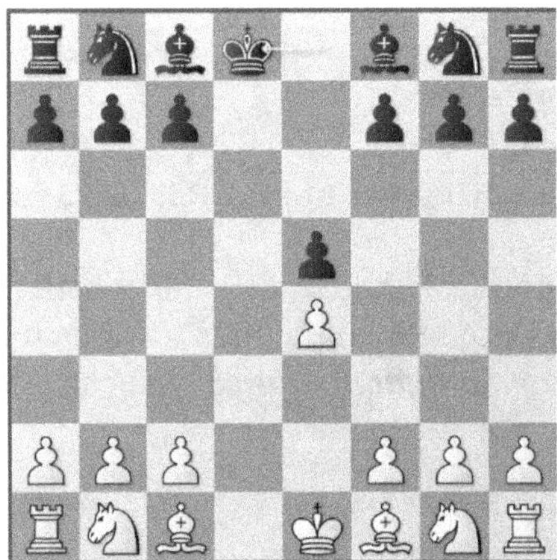

Black Lion Motif After 4...Kxd8

<u>Moves:</u> 1 e4 d6 2 d4 e5 3 dxe5 dxe5 4 Qxd8+ Kxd8 (0.40)

White has nonfatal pressure, but Black will almost certainly have familiarity, and a ton of experience with ***queenless middlegames***. This opening – a tunnel unto itself – often fall short against the tunnel, which welcomes the liquidation with full awareness that it does not yield a forced win, or even a terrible position for Black. Thanks to engines, positions like this can be tunneled all the way to a forced draw; as with all other openings, my current repertoire is a free download (as of this writing), and represents my current choice of moves for each line, which usually involves retaining a safe draw while fighting aggressively for a win. My games are also downloadable for those who wish to see this approach in practice.

Magnus Carlsen could play a line like this very easily from either side, since he tunnels through to endgames he knows almost perfectly, against players who inevitably stumble in the board fog. White's best option is 3 Nf3, converting the line into a Philidor, but this line offers much greater tree reduction, with winning chances proportional to your level of technique, something you can improve through years of constant practice akin to that of a concert pianist (a time burden I am more than happy to carry, as is any aspiring champion).

Favorable or neutral liquidation becomes a weapon unto itself, as in the QGA example that kickstarted this text. The ***Encyclopedia of Chess Middlegames*** (ECM) has a PGN file consisting of 3,001 middlegame positions, grouped thematically, that includes just about every liquidation motif and their underlying tactics and positional elements. The first step is recognizing the power of liquidation, and then aiming your play at lines that force it on favorable terms, usually involving putting pieces in each other's way, so that they lose time or space by backing off.

Very common is to see rooks traded off as they contest a single open file, with each side forced into the liquidation to avoid yielding to the other side:

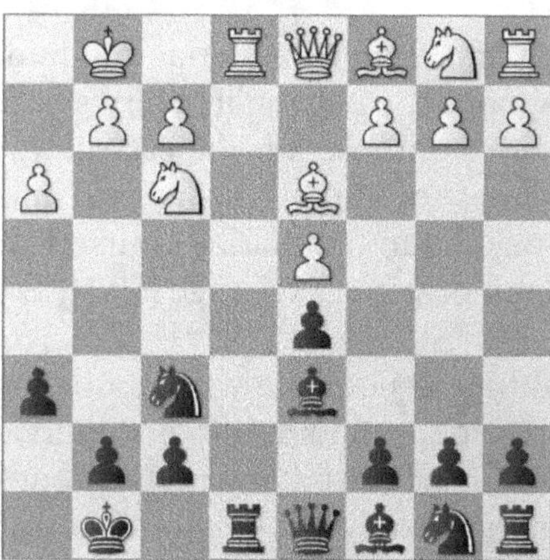

Exchange French After 8...Re8

<u>*Moves*</u>: 1 e4 e6 2 d4 d5 3 exd5 exd5 4 Nf3 Nf6 5 Bd3 Bd6 6 O-O O-O 7 h3 h6 8 Re1 Re8

While many moves are playable, 9 Rxe8+ is rated best by the silicon:

1. (0.24): 9.Rxe8+ Qxe8 10.Nc3 a6 11.Ne2 Bd7 12.Bf4 Qe7 13.Bxd6 Qxd6 14.Ng3 Qb6 15.Qc1 c5 16.dxc5 Qxc5 17.Qd2 Nc6 18.Re1 Re8 19.Rxe8+ Nxe8

2. (-0.06): 9.c3 Rxe1+ 10.Qxe1 Nc6 11.Ne5 Qe8 12.Bf4 Nxe5 13.dxe5 Nd7 14.Nd2 Nxe5 15.Bxe5 Qxe5 16.Qxe5 Bxe5 17.Re1 f6 18.Nc4 dxc4 19.Bxc4+ Be6 20.Bxe6+ Kf8

3. (-0.08): 9.Re2 Rxe2 10.Qxe2 Nc6 11.c3 Ne7 12.Ne5 Bf5 13.Bf4 Bxd3 14.Qxd3 Ne4 15.Nd2 Bxe5 16.Bxe5 Nxd2 17.Qxd2 c6 18.Bh2 Qd7 19.Qe3 Nf5

4. (-0.08): 9.Nc3 Rxe1+ 10.Qxe1 Nc6 11.Nb5 Bf8 12.a3 a6 13.Nc3 Bd6 14.Qd1 Ne7 15.Ne2 Bf5 16.Bf4 Bxd3 17.Qxd3 Bxf4 18.Nxf4 Qd6 19.Ne2 Re8 20.Re1 Nc6 21.c3 Na5

5. (-0.09): 9.a3 Rxe1+ 10.Qxe1 Nc6 11.Nc3 Ne7 12.Nb5 Bf5 13.Bxf5 Nxf5 14.Nxd6 Qxd6 15.g4 Re8 16.Qb4 Ne7 17.Qxd6 cxd6 18.Kf1 Nc6 19.Be3 h5 20.gxh5 Nxh5 21.a4 Ne7

6. (-0.12): 9.Be3 Nc6 10.a3 Ne7 11.c4 dxc4 12.Bxc4 Ned5 13.Nc3 c6 14.Qb3 Qb6 15.Nxd5 Nxd5 16.Bxd5 cxd5 17.Qxb6 axb6 18.Bd2 Bf5 19.g4 Be4 20.Nh4

7. (-0.15): 9.Na3 Rxe1+ 10.Qxe1 c6 11.c4 dxc4 12.Nxc4 Bc7 13.Nce5 Nbd7 14.Bc2 Nf8 15.Bd2 a5 16.Qe3 Be6 17.a4

8. (-0.16): 9.Bd2 Rxe1+ 10.Qxe1 Nc6 11.c4 dxc4 12.Bxc4 Bf5 13.Nc3 Qd7 14.Ne5 Bxe5 15.dxe5 Re8 16.Bb5 a6 17.Bxc6 Qxc6 18.Bf4 Ne4 19.Rd1 Nxc3 20.Qxc3 Qxc3

9. (-0.17): 9.b3 Rxe1+ 10.Qxe1 Nc6 11.Ba3 Be6 12.Bxd6 Qxd6 13.Nc3 Nb4 14.Qd2 c6 15.a4 Nxd3 16.Qxd3 Re8 17.Ne5 a6 18.Re1 Bc8 19.Re3 Qb4 20.Ne2 Ne4

Sacrificing centipawns to achieve tree reduction or liquidation is a fair trade, but giving away 0.20 for no good reason serves only to leave your opponent closer to victory, or with a reduced drawing zone for you. Contesting open lines (files or diagonals) is a good way to trade off all or most of your major pieces, as they line up to increase pressure on each side, pressure which is then best relieved through liquidation, after which the conflict peters out to a usually-drawn ending that is easily drawn by elite players, but which is still way too complicated for even strong masters to hold against players like Carlsen. With chess a forced draw, this is by far the best way to try for a win.

Weaker players are often tricked into hanging material in liquidation, or they trade down on unfavorable terms, increasing their opponent's edge with every swap. Liquidation for its own sake accomplishes little, but when done with a purpose it is the easiest way to simplify to a win or a draw. I also do not recommend giving up bishops for knights, or making other theoretically unfavorable exchanges, without a very good reason, and to familiarize yourself with the different combinations of remaining pieces after each possible minor-piece exchange (BxN, BxB, NxN, and NxB).

As with most technique, your ability to liquidate will improve naturally as you become more familiar with your opening repertoire, and need not be studied individually, though I'm sure that the **Summer of Twenty-One** (1988), which I spent studying nothing but specialized endgame books, including two weeks with Queen and Pawn endings (which often result from pawn endings after promotion, certainly aided my development. Still, I find that almost all of my improvement throughout my life (or lack thereof) has been the direct result of sharpening my repertoire. The two exceptions to this are ECM and **Domination in 2,545 Endgame Studies**, each of which gave me a strong foundation beyond the opening and to the endgame.

Prioritizing liquidation will naturally throw you into many more middlegames and endgames than you would otherwise be playing, leading to increased proficiency and smoother technique for closing out wins or holding draws. Over time, simply prioritizing liquidation and understanding its specific purpose will expand your vision to include moves which promote this, similar to how I found 3…Qd7! in the QGA line from the introduction.

Three:
Solving Trick Openings (Rating Distribution)

A relatively simple and well-known statistic among chessplayers has a dominant impact on opening play and our ratings, yet we (almost) completely ignore it. According to USCF, as of 2004, less than *one percent* of the membership was rated 2200+, a sharp dropoff even from 2100+, which has almost double the number of players, and 2000+, which checks in at 3.06 percent (the 96.94[th] percentile). At 2500, the pool drops to an infinitesimal 0.012 percent of the membership, most of whom begin playing only against each other in premier sections, round robins and invitationals. Open swisses kick the rating tires the best, however, since any holes in the repertoire will wind up in 2100-level quicksand until plugged, but once one has a working repertoire, they can "tunnel" it to a sharply decreasing opponent pool, making it easier to keep their rating afloat.

The size of your opponent pool will influence your development as a player:

◆ *Under 2200*, openings still matter (especially if you want to climb above 2200), but the large opponent pool ensures you will have every *trick* opening in the book thrown at you, and until you can solve *all* of them with heuristics, you will be stuck in *rating quicksand* that can seem eternal, but which is definitely not. It just takes seemingly *forever* to wade through what seems like an endless pile of *crap*, but again, which is not. Most players do not play through this part of their development, conclude that *openings don't matter*, and stop studying them, when doing the opposite will eventually clear this hump, for remarkably smooth sailing once one crosses into master territory.

◆ *From 2200-2700*, you'll play the correct moves, without completely understanding why, and will often live "move to move" without a purpose, making seemingly good moves almost every time, but without an overarching purpose that weaponizes the opening instead of just trying to survive. You'll also still have difficulty closing out wins, a much more difficult task than ever in the engine era.

◆ *Over 2700* is when the fun starts: your repertoire is complete, and your technique has begun to catch up. The fastest way to the top is to choose a repertoire that you won't have to change on the way up, or which does not rely on *tricks* that won't work against players rated 2400+.

Put simply, until you reach 2700, your problem is lack of technique, not your repertoire (which still might require an upgrade). Indeed, if you adopt the tunnel, you'll wind up with crushing positions that you don't know how to close out, which can be very frustrating, but at some point your technique will catch up and those games will convert to easy wins, causing your rating to make yet another quantum leap.

Each rating level has its own "crap" openings, which must be refuted before your rating will advance to the next level, and you'll get the *openings-don't-matter* lecture every step of the way until you solve each trick, only to run into a more advanced trick next time out.

I was tempted to separate this pile of crap by rating, but then realized that at my level, this is no longer necessary, but the readers will certainly notice what's being thrown at them. It has just been so long since my rating was that low that I no longer recall precisely what I had to endure, so I'll focus here instead on the more recent crap, some of which I have solved, and some of which still frustrate me, but most of which I rarely see, or can easily refute:

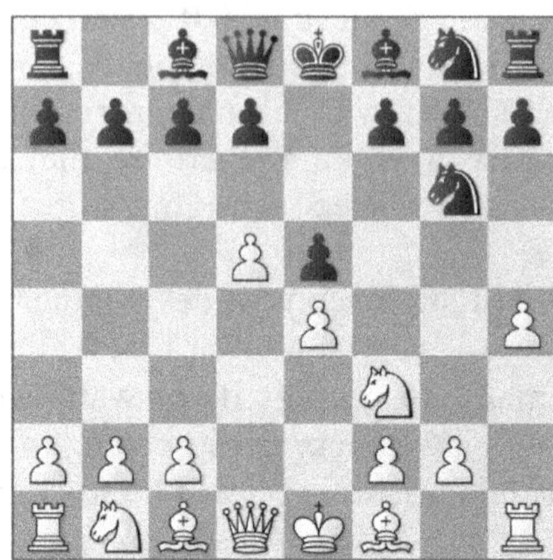

Nimzovich Defense Main Line After 5 h4

<u>Moves</u>: 1. e4 Nc6 2. d4 e5 3. d5 Nce7 4. Nf3 Ng6 5. h4

This line is "playable," (if you call *0.70 at move five* playable) but usually chosen by part-time players with no championship aspirations who can use it to reliably trick the weak, while getting suffocated by any strong opponent with decent technique. Black equalizes instantly against anything other than 2. d4, which requires extensive training and a deep understanding to play properly. In the few games where Black is tested, a 2400-rated player will simply wiggle out of the positional pressure, after which he is left with a superior pawn structure and a nice counterattack that rarely materializes against 2400+ opponents.

The result of the above is pure *gaslighting:* you're 1950, with a 3000-level repertoire, yet lose your won positions to this player, who tells you openings don't matter. Once your technique catches up, and this becomes a *rating ATM*, your previously smug opponent might lash out, or blame his losses on his "bad openings," the very ones he relied upon to get his rating, from opponents who never put him to the test.

Reality check: no player with proper technique should lose an opening up *0.70 at move five*, yet that is what will happen even to future champions on the way up, and they'll need to ignore all the condescending, *openings-don't-matter* lectures they get from players who worry only about winning now rather than years from now, much like me in 2015 when I came back to a 1500 online rating on Lichess. I've gotten this attitude every step of the way, in hundred-point increments as I solve increasingly complex…*crap*. That a player has to endure twenty years of *crap* openings on their journey to the promised land is a large reason many wind up quitting the game long before they wade through the theoretical garbage dump. Yes, I have to know how to refute lines like this to get good, but until my technique lets me do this, chess is very annoying.

Here's one from when I used to play the Sicilian Center Game:

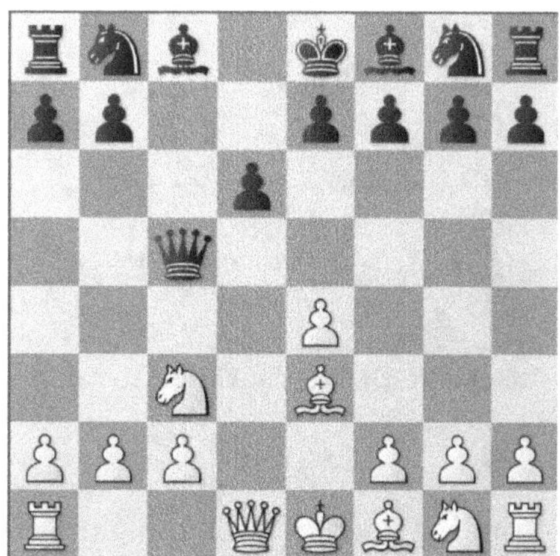

Sicilian Center Game After 5 Be3

Moves: 1 e4 c5 2 d4 d6 3 dxc5 Qa5+ 4 Nc3 Qxc5 5 Be3 (1.09)

Being up **_1.09 at move five_**, and a lot more if Black makes another error, should be enough to win easily, but White's lack of technique (on the way up) and Black's extreme familiarity makes this a **_rabbit trap_** for weak players, with Black fully aware that White is likely to fall apart, and simply ignoring the games where this doesn't happen. White is threatening Qd2 and O-O-O, followed by a queenside storm, or to even win the Black queen in some lines, but White will generally not master the refutation until he's well over 2400, which makes life hell until he gets there, since the likely outcome of this game is to lose to a 2300 from a winning position, and to have to endure the **_openings-don't-matter_** lecture from someone who relies on trick openings.

Logically, White should know that ultimately he will have technique to close out these winning positions, but most players let short-term thinking dominate, causing them to doubt the value of opening prep, because what is the point if the 2400 player just comes back to win? Simple: once your technique rises to 2400, you'll blow players like this off the board, but you'll need a lot of faith to continue training like a classical pianist and patiently developing the technique which will one day render lines like this irrelevant. At that point, the opponent pool dwindles to next to nothing, and you can tunnel almost anything against a small group of predictable players rather than the large group of talented **_randos_** who play…**_crap_**.

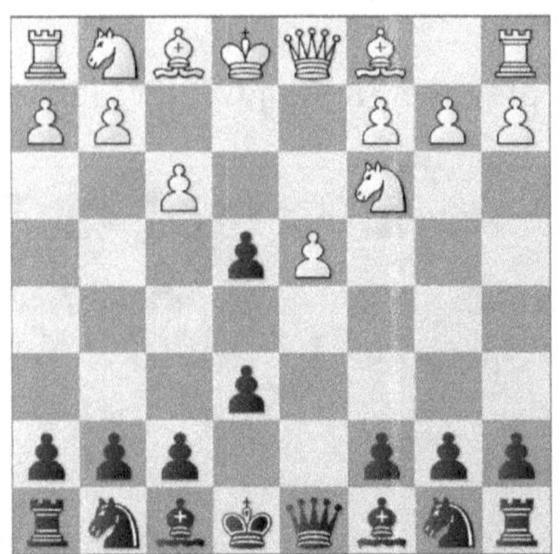

Blackmar-Diemer Sideline After 4. f3

**Moves**: 1 e4 e6 2 d4 d5 3 Nc3 dxe4 4 f3 (-0.62)

Players under 2400 are good at finding good or interesting moves in isolation, but tend not to marshal them into a complete repertoire like the tunnel. They are prone to errors like 4. f3 in the Rubinstein French, which leaves Black at **_-0.62 at move five,_** but this is just a prelude to some hall-of-fame **_crap_** after 4…Bb4!, a move not viable in the normal move order, but which is almost decisive in this one.

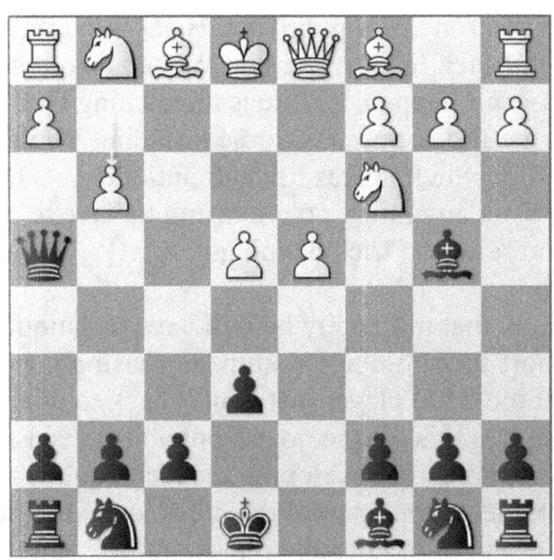

BDG Crap After 6. g3

**Moves**: 1 e4 e6 2 d4 d5 3 Nc3 dxe4 4 f3 Bb4! 5 fxe4 Qh4+ 6 g3?? (-3.88)

White could actually have stayed around -0.60 with 6 Ke2, but this **_crap_** is actually played in fast time controls (and I'm sure in some slow games, as players tend to blitz out their openings) even by masters! This may look like an easy win, but unless Black plays with absolute precision, his queen may very well not be coming home after being trapped on the back rank with all kinds of discovery and other threats from the Bf1. Generally, a quick Bd7, then either Bd6 or Nf6-Ng4 aiming at the kingside will do the trick, but make sure you rehearse this because I guarantee you **_will_** encounter it, and it **_will_** impact your rating, even if it is completely irrelevant in grandmaster play, like most of the under-2400 **_crap_**.

If, like me, you are routinely getting winning engine scores out of the opening, worry not about whether or not you convert them to wins, since that is a matter of technique. Do continue to practice and work on your middlegames (ECM) and endgames (Kasparyan) if you feel the need (do this at least twice regardless), but for the most part, ***your technique will rise naturally to match the strength of your repertoire,*** which will ultimately determine your peak. If you carve out a 2200-level repertoire with ***crap*** like the above included, don't expect to go much higher or for your technique to become stronger. On the other hand, if you copy the strongest players in the world adhering to theory, you will one day grow into that repertoire, as I have since 1986, when this became my "double stem" game (the moves I'd play against myself). I'll leave the reader with this fine example of a sound opening, later verified as such by engines:

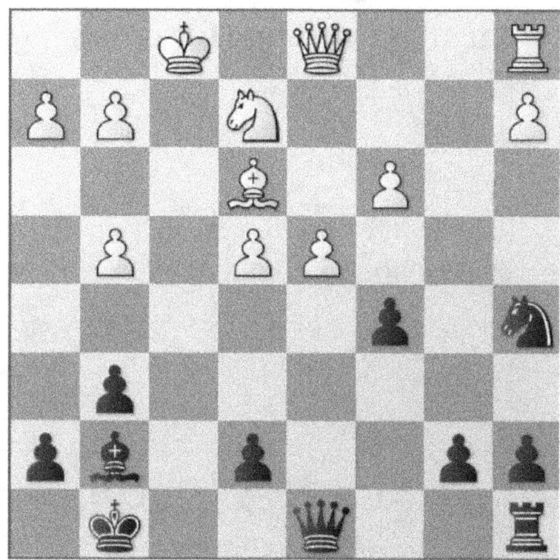

Seville Grunfeld After 14 Kxf1

Moves: 1 d4 Nf6 2 c4 g6 3 Nc3 d5 4 cxd5 Nxd5 5 e4 Nxc3 6 bxc3 Bg7 7 Bc4 c5 8 Ne2 Nc6 9 Be3 O-O 10 O-O Bg4 11 f3 Na5 12 Bxf7+ Rxf7 13 fxg4 Rxf1+ 14 Kxf1 (0.30)

This position fascinated me: why were ***these*** moves so correct that they were played from memory, almost instantly, by the two best players in the world? I wanted to see this position as Kasparov and Karpov saw it, to understand it as they did, but at the time I could barely tell apart the good moves from the bad on the way to this extended book line that had become the main line of the Grunfeld due to who was playing it. I wondered how many sound detours there were along the way, and why these moves were ruled out.

As I gained experience in the 1980s, I realized that even the world champions had a poor grasp of opening theory, because they were not ***solving*** the game like Bill Bastable, myself and others had done. This left fertile ground for improvement beyond even their level, and inspired me to embark on my journey to solve the opening, something I believe we have come closer than ever to achieving, even if "opening" variations already extend well into the middlegame and sometimes even the ending.

Rather than use ***filler*** content to lengthen this text, I have instead embraced its brevity as a sign that chess openings are deliberately overcomplicated by a coaching and publishing industry increasingly dependent on the income from chess courses and lessons, while my financial interest is the opposite, since solving 8x8 chess can only help 9x9 (for which I sell a copyrighted board design). The public is mostly to blame for this, as they search for easy answers to complex problems, but the publishers are more than happy to enable them with their silence. In the following chapters, I will cover each main tunnel line mentioned above, with analysis of both the line and any major detours you encounter along the way. It was not until I began compiling this text that I realized just how small the tunnel has made the opening move tree.

On second thought, the reader now has everything they need within this twenty-five page document to solve chess, and can refer to my free downloads for my repertoire and games, so I'm ending this project here and retiring from chess writing (for now). ***Good luck!***